CRA

Immunology and
Haematology

First and second edition authors:

Saimah Arif

Arjmand Mufti

James Griffin

Third Edition

Immunology and Haematology

Series editor
Daniel Horton-Szar
BSc (Hons), MBBS (Hons) MRCGP
Northgate Medical Practice
Canterbury
Kent, UK

Faculty advisors
Matthew Helbert
FRCP, FRCPath, PhD
Consultant Immunologist
Department of Immunology
Manchester Royal Infirmary
Manchester, UK

Caroline Shiach
BSc (Hons), MBChB, MD, FRCPath, FRCP
Consultant Haematologist
University Department of Haematology
Wythenshawe Hospital
South Manchester University Hospitals
NHS Trust
Manchester, UK

Gareth Kitchen
Medical Student
University of Manchester School of Medicine
Manchester, UK

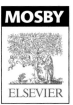

MOSBY

ELSEVIER

Edinburgh • London • New York • Oxford • Philadelphia • St Louis • Sydney • Toronto 2007

MOSBY
ELSEVIER

An imprint of Elsevier Limited

Commissioning Editor	**Andrew Miller/Alison Taylor**
Development Editor	**Kim Benson**
Project Manager	**Frances Affleck**
Senior Designer	**Sarah Russell**
Cover	**Stewart Larking**
Icon illustrations	**Geo Parkin**
Illustration Management	**Bruce Hogarth**

First edition 1998
Second edition 2003
Third edition 2007
  Reprinted 2008, 2010

ISBN-13: 978-0-7234-3418-4

British Library Cataloguing in Publication Data
A catalogue record for this book is available from the British Library

Library of Congress Cataloging in Publication Data
A catalog record for this book is available from the Library of Congress

Note
Knowledge and best practice in this field are constantly changing. As new research and experience broaden our knowledge, changes in practice, treatment and drug therapy may become necessary or appropriate. Readers are advised to check the most current information provided (i) on procedures featured or (ii) by the manufacturer of each product to be administered, to verify the recommended dose or formula, the method and duration of administration, and contraindications. It is the responsibility of the practitioner, relying on their own experience and knowledge of the patient, to make diagnoses, to determine dosages and the best treatment for each individual patient, and to take all appropriate safety precautions. To the fullest extent of the law, neither the Publisher nor the author assumes any liability for any injury and/or damage to persons or property arising out of or related to any use of the material contained in this book.
The Publisher

Writing this book has made me realize just how often immunology and haematology crop up in everyday medicine. Although they are not often taught separately in the clinical years, they are intertwined with many other of the specialities.

In *Crash Course: Immunology and Haematology* I provide up-to-date information on immunological and haematological conditions, incorporating more clinical information than previous editions.

Special effort has been made with the overview of immunology to provide a framework for immunological facts learned later to be stored.

I hope you enjoy your immunology and haematology.

Gareth Kitchen

Immunology and haematology are two of the most rapidly moving disciplines in modern medicine. In these two disciplines molecular discoveries are rapidly translated into diagnostic tests and treatments. In this Crash Course you'll read about exciting stuff such as designer drugs for leukaemia and gene therapy for immunodeficiency.

The flip side of all this progress is that these two subjects are not always taught in an up-to-date fashion and some of the newer facts get missed out. The author of this Crash Course edition, Gareth Kitchen, loves immunology and haematology. But he also loves playing rugby for Manchester. So he's found a way of conveying his interest to you and guiding you to key, up-to-date facts, so that you too can enjoy the things you love in life.

Matthew Helbert, Caroline Shiach
Faculty Advisors

More than a decade has now passed since work began on the first editions of the Crash Course series, and over 4 years since the publication of the second editions. Medicine never stands still, and the work of keeping this series relevant for today's students is an ongoing process. These third editions build upon the success of the preceding books and incorporate a great deal of new and revised material, keeping the series up to date with the latest medical research and developments in pharmacology and current best practice.

As always, we listen to feedback from the thousands of students who use Crash Course and have made further improvements to the layout and structure of the books. Each chapter now starts with a set of learning objectives, and the self-assessment sections have been enhanced and brought up to date with modern exam formats. We have also worked to integrate points of clinical relevance into the basic medical science material, which will not only add to the interest of the text but will also reinforce the principles being described.

Despite fully revising the books, we hold fast to the principles on which we first developed the series: Crash Course will always bring you all the information you need to revise in compact, manageable volumes that integrate basic medical science and clinical practice. The books still maintain the balance between clarity and conciseness, and provide sufficient depth for those aiming at distinction. The authors are medical students and junior doctors who have recent experience of the exams you are now facing, and the accuracy of the material is checked by senior faculty members from across the UK.

I wish you all the best for your future careers!

Dr Dan Horton-Szar
Series Editor

The author would like to thank Matthew Helbert, Caroline Shiach and the staff at Elsevier for their help and guidance throughout the book writing process.

Figure acknowledgements

Fig. 2.14 adapted with permission from C Janeway. Immunobiology, 4th edition. Churchill Livingstone, 1999

Figs 1.16, 1.20, 1.25, 1.28, 1.30, 2.17, 2.25 and 3.4 adapted with permission from I Roitt, D Male and I Brostoff. Immunology, 4th edition. Mosby, 1996

Figs 2.4, 4.1 and 4.14 taken with permission from A Stevens and J Lowe. Human Histology, 2nd edition. Mosby, 1997

Fig. 5.9 adapted with permission from C Haslett (editor). Davidson's Principles and Practice of Medicine, 18th edition. Churchill Livingstone, 1999

Fig. 5.19 reproduced with permission from M Makris and M Greaves. Blood in Systemic Disease. Mosby, 1997

Fig. 6.14 adapted with permission from T Gordon-Smith and J Marsh. Medicine (Haematology Part 1). The Medicine Publishing Company, 2000

Figs 7.1 and 7.4 adapted with permission from A V Hoffbrand, J Pettit and P Moss. Essential Haematology, 4th edition. Blackwell Science, 2001

Figs 8.5, 8.6, 8.7, 8.8, 8.9, 8.10, 8.11, 8.12, 8.13, 8.14, 8.15, 8.16, 8.18 and 8.20 reproduced with permission from A V Hoffbrand and J Pettit. Clinical Haematology, 2nd edition. W B Saunders, 1994

Figs in boxes on pages 13, 47, 51 and 53 reproduced with permission from R Nairn and M Helbert. Immunology for medical students, 2nd edition. Mosby, 2007

For my fiancée and family who are always there to provide support and encouragement

Contents

Active immunity Resistance to an infection or disease which develops as a result of infection or vaccination.

Adaptive immunity An immune response which is slow to respond, producing lasting immunity which can be humoral or cell mediated.

Adjuvant Substance which enhances the immune response to a vaccine.

Agglutination The process by which suspended bacteria, cells or particles clump together.

Allergen Antigenic substance which stimulates a hypersensitivity reaction.

ANCA Antinuclear cytoplasmic antibody, antibodies directed against proteinase-3 (cANCA) or against myeloperoxidase (pANCA).

Antibody Protein produced by B lymphocytes in response to the presence of an antigen.

Antigen Molecules which are recognized specifically by receptors on cells of the adaptive immune system.

Antigen-presenting cells Cells capable of presenting antigenic material to cells of the adaptive immune system.

Autoimmunity When the body's own defences are targeted against normal body cells.

Apoptosis Programmed cell death.

Atopy Possessing a genetic predisposition to an allergy.

Chemotaxis The movement of cells in response to chemicals, often to a site of infection.

Collectins A family of pattern recognition molecules, present in solution, which stimulate the innate immune system in response to a pathogen.

Complement A series of enzymatic reactions stimulated by the presence of a pathogen.

Cytokine Intercellular molecules used to transmit messages from one cell to another.

Degranulation The release of the preformed secretory granule contents by fusion with the plasma membrane.

Ecchymoses (bruises) Diffuse flat haemorrhages under the skin.

Erythropoietin A hormone, secreted by the kidney, which regulates erythropoiesis.

Haemorrhage Loss of circulating blood.

Haematocrit The relative volume of erythrocytes in the blood.

Haematoma Distinct local swelling caused by loss of blood into a muscle or subcutaneous tissue.

Haptens Small molecules which need to be bound to a large carrier molecule to be immunogenic.

HLA Human leucocyte antigen, the human form of MHC. Cell surface proteins that present antigen.

Hypersensitivity The inappropriate response of the immune system to an antigen.

Immunity A state of relative resistance to a disease.

Immunoglobulin (Ig) A protein substance secreted from plasma cells in response to infection.

Inflammation Localized response to tissue damage characterized by redness, swelling, pain, oedema and increased white cell count.

Interferon A cytokine which is targeted against viruses and intracellular bacteria.

Innate immune system Produces a non-specific response to an infection or disease.

MHC Major histocompatibility complex, a cluster of genes encoding for cell surface receptors which express antigen on the surface of cells.

Opsonin Substance that binds to a molecule to enhance its uptake by a phagocyte.

Passive immunity Passage of immunity from one individual to another.

Pathogen An organism that causes disease.

Pattern recognition molecules Molecules present either in solution or on the surface of cells which are capable of recognizing molecules characteristic of infection.

PCV Packed cell volume, measure of the proportion of blood occupied by red blood cells.

Petechiae Punctuate haemorrhages <2 mm in diameter, usually clustered.

Polymorphism Slight differences in the genetic material of individuals within a population.

Purpura Any condition with bleeding into the skin or mucous membrane.

Toll-like receptor Family of pattern recognition molecules on the cell surfaces which stimulate the innate immune system in response to a pathogen.

Urticaria Also called hives or nettle rash, characterized by an area of red inflammation and raised white bumps.

Vertical transmission Transmission of an infection from mother to fetus.

Vaccine A suspension of antigenic material injected to produce immunity against infection and disease.

IMMUNOLOGY

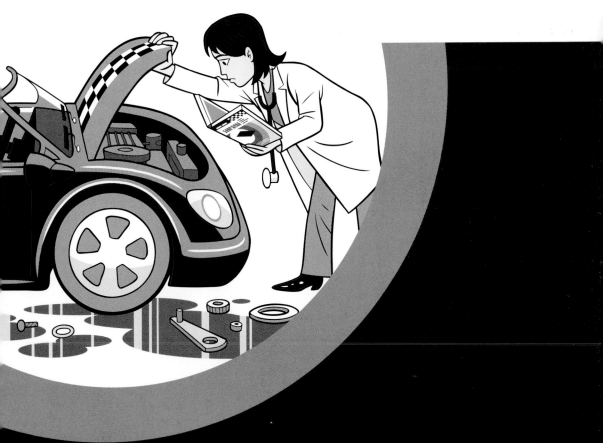

Principles of Immunology

Objectives

You should be able to:

- Have a general understanding of the immune system and its interactions
- Know the components of the innate and adaptive immune systems
- Understand how phagocytes kill pathogens
- Outline the complement cascade
- Know the functions of the differing classes of immunoglobulins
- Draw the structure and understand the functions of immunoglobulins and T cell receptors
- Understand the structure and function of MHC
- Understand the principle of genetic recombination, and how this leads to receptor diversity
- Understand the differences in the types of T helper cells and the immune responses they evoke.

AN OVERVIEW OF IMMUNOLOGY

Learning immunology is challenging, and one of those subjects that begins to make sense after the very last lecture in the module. This is because the information received in the last lecture helps you understand the first and subsequent lectures. To help with this phenomenon I start with an overview, with the purpose of providing an understanding of immunology as a whole and building a framework on which information learned later can be stored.

The function of the immune system is to protect the body from overwhelming infection. The invaders (pathogens) range from large parasitic worms living in body cavities to small viruses that can only survive inside their host cells, with bacteria, fungi and protozoans in between these two extremes of size.

These pathogens and their hosts have evolved side by side, with pathogens' increasing sophistication resulting in greater evolutionary pressure for more complex immune responses.

The first way the immune system protects against pathogens is to deny them entry through various physical barriers. These are the skin and mucous membranes that line the respiratory, gastrointestinal and reproductive tracts.

Once a pathogen has penetrated into the body, it is greeted by the human immune system. This system is divided into two forces, both of which get to work straight away: one responds quickly in a non-specific manner and the other occurs slowly and is specific to infecting organisms. These are the innate and adaptive immune systems, respectively.

The innate immune system is composed of both cellular and chemical components, the most important cellular component being the phagocyte. Phagocytes are cells that engulf foreign cells and debris (phage coming from the Greek 'to eat').

There are two types of phagocyte: the macrophage and the neutrophil. The macrophage is long lived and stationed within tissues, patrolling for the presence of trespassers. Upon contact with a pathogen (e.g. a bacterium), the macrophage engulfs it, a process known as phagocytosis. The bacterium is contained inside the macrophage, within a 'phagosome' which then fuses with a lysosome that contains enzymes and chemicals that destroy the bacterium.

Macrophages secrete chemicals called cytokines, the functions of which include attracting other cells (including short-lived neutrophils), increasing the permeability of the vascular endothelium and even increasing the production of neutrophils in the bone marrow.

3

Neutrophils act as reinforcements for the sentinel macrophages, following the trail of cytokines to the site of infection, a process called chemotaxis. Neutrophils are professional phagocytes extremely effective at killing pathogens; however, they are short lived (a failsafe to avoid excessive destruction of normal tissue) and, if the infection persists, continued secretion of cytokines will result in further mobilization of neutrophils.

Neutrophils can be recognized histologically as they have multilobed nuclei and cytoplasmic granules.

The chemical section of the innate immune system is complement. Complement comprises approximately 20 proteins that are activated through various pathways and can destroy pathogens directly through the formation of the membrane attack complex (MAC) or prepare (opsonize) them for destruction by other parts of the immune system.

The combination of phagocytes and complement systems is sufficient for dealing with most bacteria and fungi. However, certain pathogens have evolved to hide inside a host's cells where phagocytes and complement cannot reach them. Another problem with this early immune system is that a host can be infected with the same pathogen over and over again and the response has to start afresh each time.

The adaptive immune system, which evolved at about the same time as the vertebrates, has developed to combat both these flaws of the innate system. This development has led to the adaptive immune system having many more receptors for pathogenic molecules, since such receptors are formed through genetic recombination. These receptors are expressed on specialized lymphocytes called T and B cells.

T cells are able to recognize intracellular infections. This is possible as our cells evolved a method whereby the complete range of proteins within the cell is expressed as short peptides on its surface. The molecules that bind the small peptides to be expressed on the cell surface are called the major histocompatibility complex (MHC), also known as human leucocyte antigen (HLA).

B cells can release their receptors into blood and bodily secretions. These free receptors are called antibodies or immunoglobulin (Ig). The function of antibody is to flag up foreign antigens for destruction by other parts of the immune system.

Essential differences between the innate and adaptive immune systems are outlined in Fig. 1.1.

Immunity in more detail

Both the innate and adaptive immune systems comprise cellular and humoral components (Fig. 1.2).

Cytokines

Cytokines are small, secreted proteins. They act locally, via specific cell-surface receptors, as part of both the innate and adaptive immune response. Cytokines have many effects, but in general they stimulate the immune response through:

- Growth, activation and survival of various cells
- Increased production of surface molecules such as MHC.

Some important cytokines and their main actions are shown in Fig. 1.3.

Fig. 1.1 Essential differences between the innate and adaptive immune systems	
Innate immune system	**Adaptive immune system**
Provides a rapid response It is not antigen specific The response does not improve with repeated exposure	The response takes time to develop, because: • It is specific for each different antigen • Initial exposure to an antigen leaves memory cells; subsequent infections with the same antigen are therefore dealt with more quickly

Fig. 1.2 Components of the innate and adaptive immune systems

	Innate system	Adaptive system
Cellular components	Monocytes/macrophages Neutrophils Eosinophils Basophils Mast cells Natural killer cells	B cells/plasma cells T cells
Secreted components	Complement Cytokines Lysozyme Acute phase proteins Interferons	Antibody Cytokines

Fig. 1.3 Important cytokines and their actions

Cytokine	Main sources	Main actions
IL-1	Macrophages	Fever T-cell and macrophage activation
IL-2	T helper 1 cells	Growth of T cells Stimulates growth of B cells and NK cells
IL-3	T helper cells	Growth factor for progenitor haemopoietic cells
IL-4	T helper 2 cells	Activation and growth of B cells IgG1, IgE and MHC class II induction of B cells Growth and survival of T cells
IL-6	Macrophages	Lymphocyte activation Increased antibody production Fever, induces acute phase proteins
IL-8	Macrophages	Chemotactic factor for neutrophils Activates neutrophils
IL-10	T helper 2 cells Macrophages	Inhibits immune function
IL-12	Macrophages	Activates NK cells Causes CD4 T cells to differentiate into T helper 1 cells
IFN-γ	T helper 1 cells NK cells	Activation of macrophages and NK cells Produces antiviral state in neighbouring cells Increases expression of MHC class I and II molecules Inhibits T helper 2 cells
TNF-α	T helper cells Macrophages	Activates macrophages and induces nitric oxide production Proinflammatory Fever and shock
TNF-β	T helper 1 cells	Activates macrophages and neutrophils Induces nitric oxide production Kills T cells, fibroblasts and tumour cells

IL, interleukin; IFN-γ, interferon-γ; MHC, major histocompatibility complex; NK, natural killer; TNF, tumour necrosis factor.

THE INNATE IMMUNE SYSTEM

Innate defences can be classified into three main groups:

1. Barriers to infection
2. Cells
3. Serum proteins and the complement system.

Barriers to infection

Physical and mechanical

Skin and mucosal membranes act as physical barriers to the entry of pathogens. Tight junctions between cells prevent the majority of pathogens from entering the body. The flushing actions of tears, saliva and urine protect epithelial surfaces from colonization. High oxygen tension in the lungs, and body temperature, can also inhibit microbial growth.

In the respiratory tract, mucus is secreted to trap microorganisms. They are then mechanically expelled by:

- Beating cilia (mucociliary escalator)
- Coughing
- Sneezing.

Chemical

The growth of microorganisms is inhibited at acidic pH (e.g. in the stomach and vagina). Lactic acid and fatty acids in sebum (produced by sebaceous glands) maintain the skin pH between 3 and 5. Enzymes such as lysozyme (found in saliva, sweat and tears) and pepsin (present in the gut) destroy microorganisms.

Biological (normal flora)

A person's normal flora is formed when non-pathogenic bacteria colonize epithelial surfaces. Normal flora protects the host by:

- Competing with pathogenic bacteria for nutrients and attachment sites
- Production of antibacterial substances.

The use of antibiotics disrupts the normal flora and pathogenic bacteria are then more likely to cause disease.

Cells of innate immunity

The cells of the innate immune system consist of:

- Phagocytes
- Degranulating cells
- Natural killer cells.

Phagocytes

Phagocytes (macrophages and neutrophils) engulf and then destroy pathogens. Macrophages are long-lived sentinel cells stationed at likely sites of infection; upon infection they release cytokines that recruit the shorter-lived but more actively phagocytic neutrophils.

Neutrophils (for structure, see p. 97; for production, see p. 98)

Neutrophils comprise 50–70% of circulating white cells. Neutrophils arrive quickly at the site of inflammation and in the act of killing pathogens they die; in fact, dead neutrophils are the major constituent of pus. In response to tissue damage, chemicals released by macrophages and complement proteins, neutrophils migrate from the bloodstream to the site of the insult (see Chapter 2). They are phagocytes and have an important role in engulfing and killing extracellular pathogens. The process of phagocytosis and the mechanisms of killing are shown on page 7.

Neutropenic individuals are at an increased risk of serious bacterial infections. These patients should be treated early and aggressively to reduce the chance of sepsis.

Mononuclear phagocyte system

Mononuclear phagocytes comprise the other major group of phagocytic cells. Monocytes account for 5–10% of the white cell count and circulate in the blood for approximately 8 hours before migrating into the tissues, where they differentiate into macrophages; these macrophages can live for decades. Some macrophages become adapted for specific functions in particular tissues, e.g. Kupffer cells in the liver and glial cells in the brain. Monocytes also differentiate into osteoclasts and microglial cells.

In comparison to monocytes, macrophages:

- Are larger and longer-lived
- Have greater phagocytic ability

- Have a larger repertoire of lytic enzymes and secretory products.

Macrophages phagocytose and destroy their targets using similar mechanisms to neutrophils. The rate of phagocytosis can be greatly increased by opsonins such as IgG and C3b (neutrophils and macrophages have receptors for these molecules, which may be bound to the antigenic surface). Intracellular pathogens, e.g. *Mycobacterium*, can prove difficult for macrophages to kill. They are either resistant to destruction inside the phagosome or can enter the macrophage cytoplasm. For the immune system to act against these pathogens, T cell help is required.

In addition to phagocytosis, macrophages can secrete a number of compounds into the extracellular space, including cytokines (TNF and IL-1), complement components and hydrolytic enzymes. Macrophages are also able to process and present antigen in association with class II MHC molecules.

Macrophages express a wide array of surface molecules including:

- Fc-γRI–III (receptors for the Fc portion of IgG, types I–III) and complement receptors
- Receptors for bacterial constituents
- Cytokine receptors, e.g. TNF-α and interferon-γ (IFN-γ)
- MHC and B7 molecules (to activate the adaptive immune response).

Macrophages can be activated by:

- Cytokines such as IFN-γ
- Contact with complement or products of blood coagulation
- Direct contact with the target.

Following activation, macrophages become more efficient phagocytes and have increased secretory and microbicidal activity. They also stimulate the adaptive immune system by expressing higher levels of MHC class II molecules and secreting cytokines.

In comparison to neutrophils, macrophages:

- Are longer-lived (they do not die after dealing with pathogens)
- Are larger (diameter 25–50 μm), enabling phagocytosis of larger targets
- Move and phagocytose more slowly
- Exhibit a less pronounced respiratory burst
- Retain Golgi apparatus and rough endoplasmic reticulum and can therefore synthesize new proteins, including lysosomal enzymes and secretory products

- Secrete a variety of substances
- Can act as antigen-presenting cells (APCs).

Killing by phagocytes

The process of phagocytosis allows cells to engulf matter that needs to be destroyed. The cell can then digest the material in a controlled fashion before releasing the contents. The process of phagocytosis is shown in Fig. 1.4.

Microbial degradation within the phagolysosome occurs along two pathways; one requires oxygen, the other is oxygen independent.

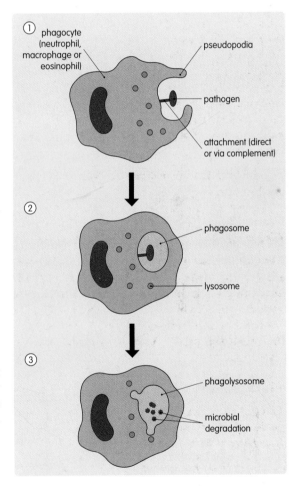

Fig. 1.4 Phagocytosis. Phagocytes sense an organism and bind it via non-specific receptors or via complement or antibody. Pseudopodia extend from the surface of the cell to surround the pathogen (1). The pseudopodia fuse around the organism, producing a vesicle known as a phagosome (2). Lysosomes fuse with the phagosome to form phagolysosomes (3). Chemicals within the lysosome, and other granules that fuse with the phagolysosome, lead to degradation of the organism. The microbial products are then released.

Oxygen-independent degradation Neutrophil granules contain several antimicrobial agents including:

- Lysozyme (splits peptidoglycan)
- Lactoferrin and reactive nitrogen intermediates (which complex with, and deprive pathogens of, iron)
- Proteolytic enzymes (degrade dead microbes)
- Defensins, cathepsin G and cationic proteins (damage microbial membranes).

Oxygen-dependent degradation

$$2O_2^{\bullet -} + 2H^+ \rightarrow H_2O_2 + O_2$$
$$O_2^{\bullet -} + H_2O_2 \rightarrow OH^{\bullet -} + OH^{\bullet -} + O_2$$
$$H_2O_2 + Cl^- \rightarrow OCl^{\bullet -} + H_2O \text{ (catalysed by}$$
myeloperoxidase)
$$OCl^{\bullet -} + \text{amine} \rightarrow \text{chloramines}$$

Hypochlorous acid (HOCl) and chloramines are longer-lived than the other oxidizing agents and are probably the most important target killing compounds in vivo. If a target cannot be easily phagocytosed, there may be extracellular release of granule contents, causing tissue damage.

Natural killer (NK) cells

NK cells do not require T cell help to kill pathogens, although they are more effective when T helper cells secrete IFN-γ. NK cells utilize cell-surface receptors to identify virally modified or cancerous cells. One set of receptors activates NK cells, initiating killing; others inhibit the cells:

- Activating receptors include calcium-binding C-lectins, which recognize certain cell-surface carbohydrates. Because these carbohydrates are present on the surface of normal host cells, a system of inhibitory receptors acts to prevent killing
- Killer inhibitor receptors (KIRs), members of the immunoglobulin gene superfamily, are specific for class I MHC molecules. Human NK cells also express an inhibitory receptor (a heterodimer CD94:NKG2) that detects non-classical class I molecules.

NK cells can also destroy antibody-coated target cells irrespective of the presence of MHC molecules, a process known as antibody-dependent cell-mediated cytotoxicity. This occurs because killing is initiated by cross-linking of receptors for the Fc portion of IgG1 and IgG3.

NK cells are not clonally restricted, have no memory and are not very specific in their action. They induce apoptosis in target cells (Fig. 1.5) by:

- Ligation of FAS or TNF receptors on the target cells (NK cells produce TNF and exhibit FASL). This initiates a sequence of caspase recruitment and activation, resulting in apoptosis
- Degranulation by NK cells, which releases perforins and granzymes. Perforin molecules

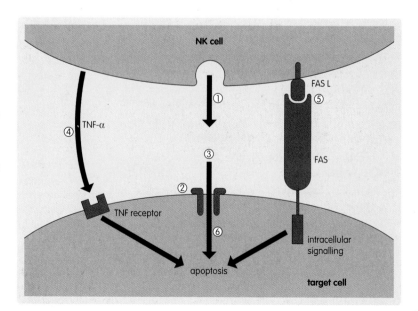

Fig. 1.5 Mechanism of killing by natural killer (NK) cells (1). Activation of NK cells in the absence of an inhibitory signal results in degranulation (2). Perforins form a pore in the target cell, allowing entry of granzymes (3). TNF produced by NK cells acts on the target's cell receptors (4). FASL interacts with target cell FAS (5). Intracellular signalling from FAS, TNF receptors and granzymes results in apoptosis (6).

---

insert into and polymerize within the target cell membrane. This forms a pore through which granzymes can pass. Granzyme B then initiates apoptosis from within the target cell cytoplasm.

Mast cells and basophils (for structure, see p. 99)

Mast cells and basophils have similar functions but are found in different locations; basophils comprise <1% of circulating white cells, whereas mast cells are resident in the tissues. This has led to the theory that mast cells are a population of differentiated basophils.

High concentrations of mast cells are found close to blood vessels in connective tissue, skin and mucosal membranes. The two types of mast cell—mucosal and connective tissue—differ in their tissue distribution, protease content and secretory profiles.

Mast cells function by discharging their granule contents. Degranulation is triggered by cross-linking of high-affinity receptors for the Fc portion of IgE (Fig. 1.6). Cross-linkage results in an influx of calcium ions into the cell, which induces release of pharmacologically active mediators from granules (Fig. 1.7). Mast cell activation releases leukotrienes, which attract eosinophils to the site of worm infection. This plays an important role in the development of an episode of a type I hypersensitivity, with the mast cells and basophils providing the early phase response and the eosinophils mediating the late phase response. This is important in allergic responses (type I hypersensitivity reactions, see p. 39).

Eosinophils (for structure, see p. 99)

Eosinophils comprise 1–3% of circulating white cells and are found principally in tissues. They are derived from the colony-forming unit for granulocytes, erythrocytes, monocytes and megakaryocytes (CFU-GEMM) haematopoietic precursor and their maturation is similar to that of the neutrophil (see p. 98). They are important in the defence against parasites and cause damage by extracellular degranulation. Their granules contain major basic protein, cationic protein, peroxidase and perforin-like molecules. The peroxidase generates hypochlorous acid, major basic protein damages the parasite's outer surface (as well as host tissues) and cationic protein acts as a neurotoxin, damaging the parasite's nervous tissue.

Soluble proteins

The soluble proteins that contribute to innate immunity (Fig. 1.8) can be divided into antimicrobial serum agents and proteins produced by cells of the immune system.

Acute phase proteins

The acute phase response is a systemic reaction to infection or tissue injury, where macrophages release cytokines IL-1, IL-6 and TNF; these cytokines reach the liver through the circulation. The liver responds by increasing its production of certain plasma proteins. These so-named acute phase proteins (APPs) are:

- C-reactive protein
- Serum amyloid A
- Complement components
- Fibrinogen
- α_1-Antitrypsin
- Caeruloplasmin
- Haptoglobulin.

The change in plasma concentration is accompanied by fever, leucocytosis, thrombocytosis, catabolism of muscle proteins and fat deposits. Synthesis of

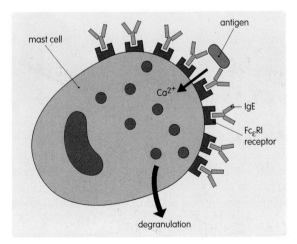

Fig. 1.6 Activation of mast cells by immunoglobulin E (IgE). IgE, produced by plasma cells, binds via its Fc domain to receptors on the mast cell surface. Cross-linking of these receptors by an antigen causes an influx of calcium ions (Ca^{2+}) into the cell. Calcium ions cause a rapid degranulation of inflammatory mediators from the mast cell.

Fig. 1.7 Mast cell mediators and their actions

Mediator			Action
Primary	Histamine		Increased capillary permeability, vasodilatation, smooth muscle contraction
	Serotonin		Increased capillary permeability, vasodilatation, smooth muscle contraction, platelet aggregation
	Heparin		Anticoagulation (see p. 119), modulates tryptase
	Proteases	Tryptase	Activates complement (C3)
		Chymase	Increased mucus secretion
	Eosinophil chemotactic factor		Chemotactic (cells move towards site of production) for eosinophils
	Neutrophil chemotactic factor		Chemotactic for neutrophils
	Acid hydrolases		Degradation of extracellular matrix
	Platelet-activating factor		Platelet aggregation and activation, increased capillary permeability, vasodilatation, chemotactic for leucocytes, neutrophil activation
Secondary	Leukotrienes (C_4, D_4, B_4)		Vasodilatation, smooth muscle contraction, mucus secretion, chemotactic for neutrophils
	Prostaglandins (D_2)		Vasodilatation, smooth muscle contraction, chemotactic for neutrophils, potentiation of other mediators
	Bradykinin		Increased capillary permeability, vasodilatation, smooth muscle contraction, stimulation of pain nerve endings
	Cytokines		Various

Mast cells contain many preformed (primary) mediators that are stored in granules. They can also synthesize new (secondary) mediators when they are activated.

APPs is enhanced by cytokines secreted by macrophages and endothelial cells. The two main APPs are C-reactive protein (CRP) and serum amyloid A (SAA).

The extent of the rise in the plasma concentration of different APPs varies:

- Increased 50% above normal levels: caeruloplasmin
- Increased several fold above normal levels: α_1-glycoprotein, α_1-proteinase inhibitor, haptoglobulin, fibrinogen
- 100–1000-fold increase: CRP, SAA.

The concentration of other plasma proteins, most notably albumin and transferrin, falls.

C-reactive protein

Levels of CRP rise within hours of tissue injury or infection. The actions of CRP are outlined in Fig. 1.8. CRP elevation can be slight (e.g. cerebrovascular accident), moderate (e.g. myocardial infarction) or marked (e.g. bacterial infections).

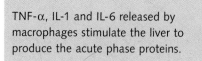

TNF-α, IL-1 and IL-6 released by macrophages stimulate the liver to produce the acute phase proteins.

Serum amyloid A

SAA levels rise within hours of tissue injury or infection. SAA may function as an opsonin. Persistent elevation of SAA can lead to its deposition in tissues in amyloidosis (see p. 109).

Erythrocyte sedimentation rate

The erythrocyte sedimentation rate (ESR) is an index of the acute phase response. It is especially representative of the concentration of fibrinogen and α-globulins. Elevated fibrinogen levels cause red cells to form stacks (rouleaux), which sediment more rapidly than individual blood cells.

Fig. 1.8 The soluble proteins of innate immunity

	Protein	Notes
Secreted agents	Lysozyme	Bactericidal enzyme in mucus, saliva, tears, sweat and breast milk Cleaves peptidoglycan in the cell wall
Innate antimicrobial serum agents	Lactoferrin	Iron-binding protein that competes with microorganisms for iron, an essential metabolite
	Complement	Group of ~20 proenzymes Activation leads to an enzyme cascade, the products of which enhance phagocytosis and mediate cell lysis Alternative pathway can be activated by non-specific mechanism
	Mannan-binding lectin	Activates the complement system
	C-reactive protein	Acute phase protein, produced by the liver Serum concentration rises >100-fold in tissue-damaging infections Binds C-polysaccharide cell wall component of bacteria and fungi Activates complement via classical pathway Opsonizes for phagocytosis
Proteins produced by cells of the innate system	Interferon-α Interferon-β	Produced by virally infected cells Induces a state of viral resistance in neighbouring cells by: • Inducing genes that will destroy viral DNA • Inducing MHC class I expression
	Interferon-γ	Mainly produced by activated NK cells Activates NK cells and macrophages

MHC, major histocompatibility complex; NK, natural killer.

In chronic inflammation, high CRP and ESR persist. The resulting catabolism of muscle and fat may lead to severe weight loss.

The acute phase response

The acute phase response provides us with chemical markers of inflammation that can be measured. In a child presenting with abdominal pain a CRP can aid the clinician in their diagnosis. A normal CRP can allow more conservative management whereas a raised CRP would indicate an inflammatory response and necessitate urgent treatment, such as surgery in differentiating the abdominal pain in constipation from that of appendicitis.

ESR takes more time than CRP to become elevated, and is a useful marker measured in chronic inflammatory diseases.

The complement system

The complement system—so-called because scientists compared its *complementary* actions to the function of antibody—is, in fact, much older in evolutionary terms than antibody and is equally important.

Complement is a collection of over 20 serum proteins that are always at high levels in the blood of the healthy individual. The complement system may seem complex with all the alphanumerical naming and active and inactive components. Thinking about it simply, it is a system that has three methods of activating a common pathway, which in turn has three results or effectors. The reason for the large number of proteins is to allow amplification; many of the components of complement are proenzymes that, when cleaved, activate more complement.

The three pathways that activate the complement system are the classical, the alternative and the lectin. All pathways result in the activation of the complement component C3 to C3 convertase. An overview of the complement system is given in Fig. 1.9.

Fig. 1.9 Overview of the complement system. Cell lysis by complement is due to formation of the membrane attack complex (MAC). This is formed when C5b, C6, C7, C8 and C9 bind together to form a 10-nm pore in the cell surface. MASP, mannan-binding lectin associated serine protease.

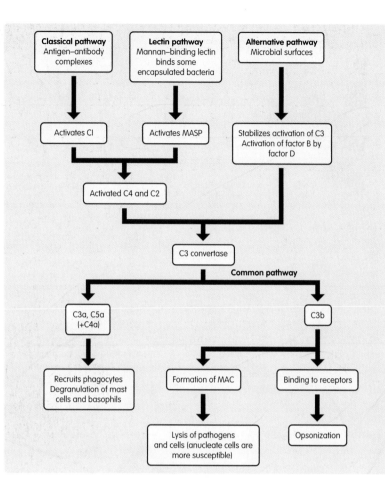

The classical pathway

The classical pathway was discovered first and involves the activation of complement by the Fc portion of antibody. IgM is particularly good at activating complement as it is a pentamer (has five Fc portions):

- Fc activates C1
- C1 activates C2 and C4
- C2 and C4 activate C3 (C3 convertase).

The alternative pathway

C3 is an unstable molecule and without inhibition spontaneously breaks down to the very reactive C3b; C3b reacts to two common chemical functional groups, the amino and hydroxyl groups. C3b is therefore neutralized quickly by water. However, with many pathogens made up of proteins and carbohydrates that contain these functional groups, C3b attaches to the pathogen and is not broken down. C3b then reacts with more complement components to form C3bBb; this is C3 convertase.

The lectin pathway

Mannan-binding lectin (MBL), which is normally found in serum, binds to MBL-associated serine proteases (MASP). This complex bears structural homology to the C1 complex. When MBL binds to carbohydrate on the surface of bacteria, MASP is activated. MASP then acts on C4 and C2 to generate the C3 convertase of the classical pathway.

C3 convertase

With the production of C3 convertase, all three pathways converge. C3 convertase has enzymatic effects against C3 and enables the production of large quantities of C3b, thus producing a major amplification step in the complement pathway.

Effectors of complement

C5 is cleaved into C5a and C5b, and C5b triggers the activation of C6–C9. These form the membrane attack complex (MAC). The MAC attacks pathogens by inserting a hole in their cell membrane; the

Fig. 1.10 Functions of complement

Function	Notes
Cell lysis	Insertion of MAC causes lysis of Gram-negative bacteria Nucleated cells are more resistant to lysis because they endocytose MAC
Inflammation	C3a, C4a, C5a cause degranulation of mast cells and basophils C3a and C5a are chemotactic for neutrophils
Opsonization	Phagocytes have C3b receptors, which means that they are able to phagocytose antigen coated in C3b
Solubilization and clearance of immune complexes	Complement prevents immune complex precipitation and solubilizes complexes that have already been precipitated Complexes coated in C3b bind to CR1 on red blood cells The complexes are then removed in the spleen

MAC, membrane attack complex.

pathogen then dies via osmotic lysis. The MAC appears to be the only way the immune system has of killing one family of bacteria, the *Neisseria* (a family that includes meningococcus and gonococcus).

The cleaved fragments C3b and C5b are anaphylotoxins which are chemoattractant for other immune cells which follow the concentration gradient to the infection. Complement also opsonizes bacteria as macrophages have receptors for C3b.

These functions are summarized in Fig. 1.10.

Inhibitors of complement

As we have seen, complement can activate spontaneously through the alternative pathway. Complement is regulated by inhibitory molecules which are necessary to prevent complement-mediated damage of healthy cells. There are nine complement inhibitors which act at various levels throughout the pathway:

- Membrane cofactor protein, complement receptor type 1, C4b-binding protein and factor H: these prevent assembly of C3 convertase
- Decay accelerating factor: this accelerates decay of C3 convertase
- C1 inhibitor: inhibits C1
- Factor I and membrane cofactor protein: cleave C3b and C4b
- CD59 (protectin): prevents the formation of the membrane attack complex (MAC).

Hereditary angioedema

Deficiency in even one of these inhibitory components can result in significant disease. For example, deficiency in C1 inhibitor results in hereditary angioedema (HAE; see photograph), a condition where there is activation of the classical pathway with minimal stimulation. This is of particular significance if the stimulation is in the larynx as it can lead to uncontrolled swelling. This laryngeal oedema can obstruct the airway and without infusion of C1 inhibitor can prove fatal.

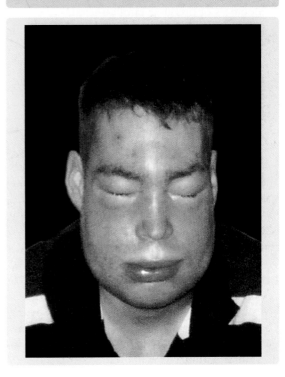

RECOGNITION MOLECULES

We have already come across the recognition molecules MBL and C1q in the complement system. These are found in solution in the serum and are classified as collectins, being composed of collagen-like and lectin portions. Lectins are any protein that binds sugar molecules, usually on the surface of bacteria, e.g. MBL binds to the sugar mannose.

Another group of non-specific receptors for pathogens are the Toll-like receptors, transmembrane receptors found on antigen-presenting cells. Each Toll-like receptor recognizes a different type of pathogenic molecule, e.g. TLR4 binds lipopolysaccharide present in bacterial membranes and also fungi. Activation stimulates the production of cytokines and co-stimulatory molecules which facilitate an adaptive immune response.

The immunoglobulin domain

B and T cell surface receptors are members of the immunoglobulin gene superfamily. Genes in this family code for proteins composed of motifs called immunoglobulin domains. All molecules in the immunoglobulin superfamily extend from the surface of cells. They are flexible and include specialist domains; the antigen receptor site on B cell receptors is an example.

Members of this gene family include:

- Immunoglobulin (B cell receptor)
- T cell receptor
- MHC molecules
- T cell accessory molecules such as CD4
- Certain adhesion molecules, e.g. ICAM-1, ICAM-2 and VCAM-1.

Each domain is approximately 110 amino acids in length. The polypeptide chain in each domain is folded into seven or eight antiparallel beta strands. The strands are arranged to form two opposing sheets, linked by a disulphide bond and hydrophobic interactions. This compact structure is called the immunoglobulin fold.

Structure of B and T cell surface antigen receptors

Structure of immunoglobulin

The B cell surface receptor is a membrane-bound immunoglobulin (mIg) molecule. mIg recognizes the conformational structure (shape) of antigenic

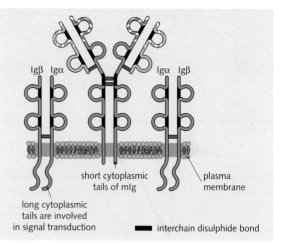

Fig. 1.11 Structure of the B cell surface receptor. Membrane-bound immunoglobulin is non-signalling. It associates with two Ig-α/Ig-β heterodimers (members of the immunoglobulin gene superfamily), which have long cytoplasmic domains capable of transducing a signal.

epitopes. Ig is composed of two light and two heavy chains. In the B cell receptor (Fig. 1.11), mIg associates with two Ig-α/Ig-β dimers (members of the immunoglobulin gene superfamily). Signal transduction through the mIg is thought to be mediated by the Ig-α/Ig-β heterodimers.

Ig is also secreted by plasma cells (see p. 20). The extracellular portion of mIg is identical in structure to secretory Ig. mIg differs from secreted Ig (sIg) because it has transmembrane and cytoplasmic portions that anchor it to the membrane. Different Ig classes can be expressed on the same B cell and may indicate the stage of development of the B cell, e.g. a mature, but antigenically unchallenged, B cell expresses both mIgM and mIgD. The antigenic specificity of all of the mIg molecules expressed on any given B cell is the same.

Antigen recognition by T cells differs from antigen recognition by B cells:

- T cells recognize antigen only when it is associated with a molecule of the MHC
- T cells recognize peptide fragments of an antigen in association with MHC molecules; these fragments of antigen are processed by APCs before they are presented to the T cell.

The T cell surface antigen receptor consists of the T cell receptor (TCR) associated with CD3. The TCR is a heterodimer, comprising α- and β-chains, or γ- and δ-chains. Approximately 95% of T cells express αβ-receptors. The TCR is structurally similar to the immunoglobulin Fab region (see p. 21). Each chain comprises two immunoglobulin domains, one variable and one constant, linked by a disulphide bond. As in the variable domains of immunoglobulin, three variable regions on each chain combine to form the antigen-binding site.

CD3 is made up of three polypeptide dimers, consisting of four or five different peptide chains. The dimers are γε, δε and ζζ (found in 90% of CD3 molecules) or ζη. The γ-, δ- and ε-chains are members of the Ig gene superfamily. The TCR recognizes and binds antigen, and CD3, functionally analogous to the Ig-α/Ig-β heterodimer in B cells, is involved in signal transduction (Fig. 1.12).

The major histocompatibility complex (MHC)

Major histocompatibility complex (MHC) is a generic term for a group of molecules produced by higher vertebrate species. The human leucocyte antigen (HLA) system is the human MHC.

The MHC genes

A complete set of MHC alleles inherited from one parent is referred to as a haplotype.

MHC genes exhibit a high degree of polymorphism, i.e. they exhibit considerable diversity (there are more than 100 identified alleles for human leucocyte antigen B (HLA-B)). This means that most individuals will be heterozygous at most MHC loci and that any two randomly selected individuals are very unlikely to have identical HLA alleles. Diversity of the MHC increases the chance that a person will be able to mount an adaptive response against a pathogen. The genetic loci are tightly linked, so that one set is inherited from each parent. The genes are divided into three regions, each region encoding one of the three classes of the MHC: class I, class II and class III (Fig. 1.13). The MHC alleles exhibit codominance, which means that both alleles are expressed.

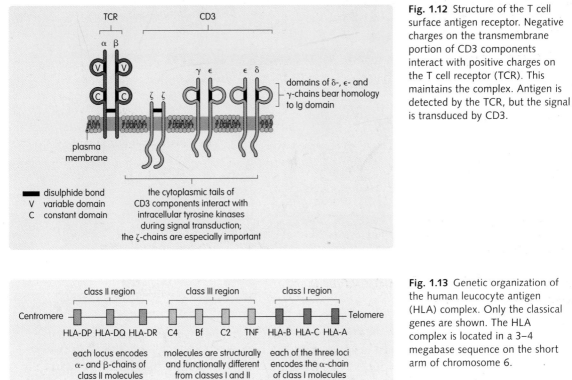

Fig. **1.12** Structure of the T cell surface antigen receptor. Negative charges on the transmembrane portion of CD3 components interact with positive charges on the T cell receptor (TCR). This maintains the complex. Antigen is detected by the TCR, but the signal is transduced by CD3.

Fig. **1.13** Genetic organization of the human leucocyte antigen (HLA) complex. Only the classical genes are shown. The HLA complex is located in a 3–4 megabase sequence on the short arm of chromosome 6.

Structure and function of the MHC

Class I and class II MHC molecules are glycoproteins expressed on the cell surface and consist of cytoplasmic, transmembrane and extracellular portions (Fig. 1.14). Both class I and class II molecules exhibit broad specificity in their binding of peptide. The polymorphism of the MHC is largely concentrated in the peptide binding cleft. A summary of the differences between class I and class II MHC molecules is shown in Fig. 1.15.

MHC restriction

T cells are only able to recognize antigen in the context of self-MHC molecules (self-MHC restriction). CD8[+] T cells recognize antigen only in association with class I MHC molecules (class I MHC

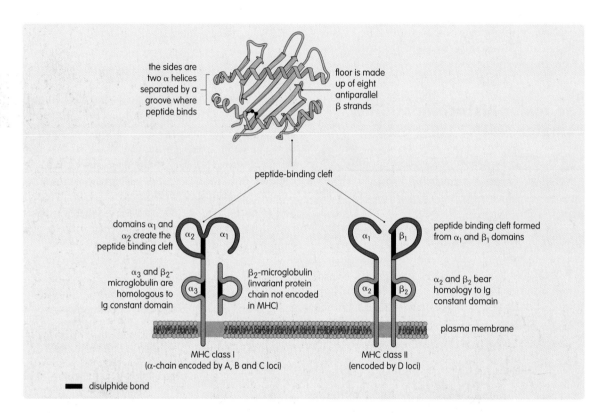

Fig. 1.14 Structure of class I and class II major histocompatibility molecules (MHC). The peptide binding cleft of a class I molecule is also shown as seen from above.

Fig. 1.15 Differences between class I and class II major histocompatibility molecules		
	Class I	**Class II**
Size of bound peptide	8–9 amino acids	13–18 amino acids (binding cleft more open)
Peptide from	Cytosolic antigen	Intravesicular or extracellular antigen
Expressed by	All nucleated cells, especially T cells, B cells, macrophages, other antigen-presenting cells, neutrophils	B cells, macrophages, other antigen-presenting cells, epithelial cells of the thymus, activated T cells
Recognized by	CD8[+] T cells	CD4[+] T cells

restricted). CD4+ cells recognize antigen only in association with class II MHC molecules (class II MHC restricted).

Antigen processing and presentation

MHC molecules do not present whole antigen, the antigen being degraded into peptide fragments before binding can occur. There are different pathways of antigen processing for class I and class II MHC; these pathways are summarized in Fig. 1.16.

Professional APCs process and present antigen to CD4+ T cells in association with class II molecules. These cells express high levels of class II MHC molecules. Professional APCs include:

- Dendritic cells, including Langerhans' cells
- Macrophages
- B cells.

Structure and function of CD4 and CD8

CD4 and CD8 are 'accessory' molecules that play an important role in the T cell–antigen interaction. CD4 and CD8 have two important functions:

- They bind MHC class II and class I molecules, respectively, thereby strengthening the T cell–antigen interaction
- They function as signal transducers.

The role of CD4 and CD8 in antigen–receptor binding is shown in Fig. 1.17.

GENERATION OF ANTIGEN RECEPTOR DIVERSITY

Scientists know that there are approximately 20^8 possible antigens, each requiring a corresponding

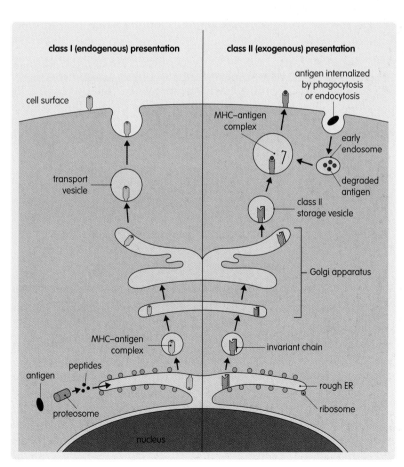

Fig. 1.16 Routes of antigen processing. Class I molecules present endogenous antigens. Cytosolic antigen is degraded by proteosomes and transported into the rough endoplasmic reticulum (ER), where peptides are loaded onto class I molecules. The MHC–peptide complex is transported via the Golgi apparatus to the cell surface. Class II molecules present exogenous antigens that have been phago- or endocytosed into intracellular vesicles. The MHC molecule is transported from the rough ER to the vesicle by the invariant chain (Ii). It is displaced from the MHC molecule by processed antigen, which is then presented at the cell surface. MHC, major histocompatibility complex.

Fig. 1.17 The role of CD4 and CD8 in T cell receptor (TCR)–major histocompatibility complex (MHC) antigen interaction. CD4 or CD8 is closely associated with the TCR complex. They bind MHC in a restricted fashion (CD8 to class I only, CD4 to class II only). Binding is antigen independent and strengthens the bond between TCR and a complementary peptide–MHC complex. Molecules associated with CD4 or CD8 are then able to transduce a signal.

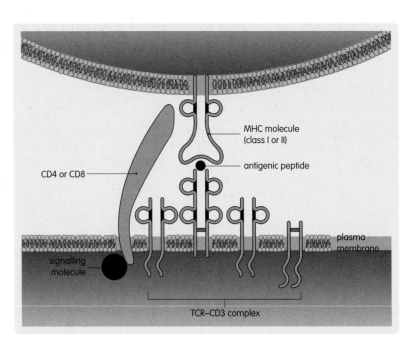

receptor. The human genome contains only 30,000 genes and so each receptor cannot be coded by a single gene. Instead this diversity is achieved by genetic recombination, a process where segments of information are cut and pasted from the gene.

T cell receptor and immunoglobulin are the only genes to undergo genetic recombination.

Rearrangement of gene segments allows antibodies with an immense variety of specificity to be produced from a relatively small amount of DNA.

Genetic rearrangements

Before genetic recombination occurs, we say the gene segments are in germline configuration. Rearrangement only occurs in the variable domain (those that code for the active site) as the other segments of the receptor remain constant. Each variable domain is encoded by a random combination of one of each of the V, D (heavy chain only) and J exons. Following genetic rearrangement, one exon remains which codes for a variable domain. The C exons encode the constant regions. Heavy-chain C gene segments are clusters of exons, each of which encodes either a domain or a hinge region of the constant region.

Following rearrangement, the clonal progeny of each B cell will produce Ig of a single specificity. Rearrangement is completed and functional Ig chains are produced before the B cell encounters antigen (Fig. 1.18). The presence of multiple V, D (heavy chain only) and J gene segments, and the apparently random selection of these segments, generates considerable diversity, which can be calculated (Fig. 1.19).

A similar process occurs in T cells: α- and γ-chain variable domains have V and J segments; β- and δ-chains have V, D and J segments.

Junctional diversity

The formation of junctions between the various gene segments produces an opportunity for increased diversity, where nucleotides are added or subtracted at random to form the joining segments.

Junctional flexibility and N-nucleotide addition

When exons are spliced, there are slight variations in the position of segmental joining. In addition, up to 15 nucleotides can be added to the D–J and the V–DJ joints. This occurs only in heavy chains and is catalysed by terminal deoxynucleotidyl transferase (TdT).

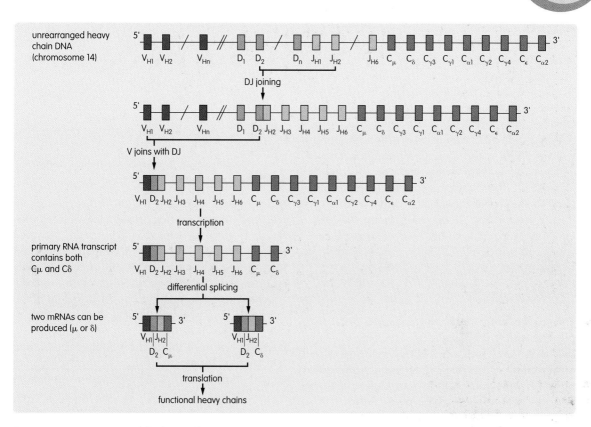

Fig. 1.18 Rearrangement of the heavy chain is similar to that of the light chain, although the join between D and J segments occurs first. In an unstimulated B cell, the heavy-chain mRNA that is transcribed contains both the $C\mu$ and $C\delta$ segments. The mRNA can be differentially spliced such that both IgM and IgD will be produced. They will both exhibit the same antigen binding specificity.

Fig. 1.19 Calculation of antibody diversity

	Number of combinations		
Mechanism of diversity	**κ light chain**	**λ light chain**	**Heavy chain**
Random joining of gene segments	$100 \times 5 = 500$	$100 \times 6 = 600$	$75 \times 30 \times 6 = 13{,}500$
Random chain associations	$(500 + 600) \times 13{,}500 = 1.5 \times 10^7$		

Given the fact that light chain can associate with any heavy chain, and from the number of gene segments present in germline DNA, it is possible to calculate the number of different molecules that can be produced. The extent of the contribution of junctional flexibility, N-nucleotide addition and somatic hypermutation is not known but will be significant.

Both junctional flexibility and N-nucleotide addition can disrupt the reading frame, leading to non-functional rearrangements. However, formation of productive rearrangements increases antibody diversity. The V–J, V–DJ and VD–J joints fall within the antigen-binding region of the variable domain. Therefore, diversity generated at these joints will impact on the antigen specificity of the Ig molecule.

Somatic hypermutation

Somatic hypermutation is a process that increases the affinity of antibody for its antigen and is also called affinity maturation. B cells that are dividing by mitosis to increase in number in order to combat infection are allowed to undergo mutation in their variable domain (the only cells in the body permitted to do so). Some mutations decrease the antibody's specificity for the antigen and apoptosis is stimulated in these cells; others result in antibody of increased specificity—these are positively selected for. Antibodies produced later in the primary immune response, and in the secondary immune response, will therefore have an increased affinity for antigen.

The TCR does not exhibit somatic hypermutation. This is probably because T cells do not recognize self-peptides, recognizing only self-MHC. Diversity is generated only in developing T cells, which can be deleted if they are either self-reactive or non-functional.

Class switching

This is the process whereby a single B cell can produce different classes of Ig that have the same specificity. The mechanism is not well understood but involves 'switch sites'—DNA sequences located upstream from each heavy chain C gene segment (except C_δ). Possible mechanisms include:

- Differential splicing of the primary transcript (see Fig. 1.18)
- A looping out and deletion of intervening heavy chain C gene segments (and introns)
- Exchange of C gene segments between chromosomes.

This process underlies the class switch from IgM in the primary response to IgG, IgA or IgE in the secondary response. Cytokines are important in controlling the switch.

THE ADAPTIVE IMMUNE SYSTEM

Recognition molecules and their diversity are important for the generation of a specific, adaptive immune response. The adaptive immune response can be humoral or cell-mediated.

HUMORAL IMMUNITY

B cells and antibody production

The humoral immune response is brought about by antibodies, which are particularly efficient at eliminating extracellular pathogens. Antigen can be cleared from the host by a variety of effector mechanisms, which are dependent on antibody class or isotype (see p. 23):

- Activation of complement, leading to lysis or opsonization of the microorganism
- Antibody-dependent cell-mediated cytotoxicity (ADCC)
- Neutralization of bacterial toxins and viruses
- Mucosal immunity (IgA-mediated).

Activated and differentiated B cells, known as plasma cells, produce antibodies. An overview of B cell activation is given in Fig. 1.20. B cells are activated within follicles found in secondary lymphoid structures, e.g. lymph nodes and spleen. B cells become activated only if they encounter specific antigen. During proliferation, variable regions of the immunoglobulin genes undergo somatic hypermutation (see p. 19). This process occurs in the germinal centre of the follicle. Follicular dendritic cells present antigen, to which the B cells with the highest affinity will bind. This causes the expression of bcl-2, which prevents B cells undergoing apoptosis. Therefore, the highest-affinity clones are positively selected. In order for B cells to produce antibody, they require help from T cells. Activated T helper cells provide the help needed by producing cytokines (IL-2, IL-4, IL-5, IL-6). This acts as a further method of regulation within the immune system, as both B cells and T cells need exposure to the offending antigen in order for a response to be evoked. In addition, as self-reactive T cells are deleted in the thymus, the chance of autoimmunity is reduced. An overview of clonal selection of B cells is given in Fig. 1.21.

T-cell-dependent and T-cell-independent antigens

The process shown in Fig. 1.20 illustrates the need for T cells in the activation of a humoral response. The antigens that trigger this process are therefore known as T-cell-dependent antigens. Not all antigens require T cells to produce an antibody response. T-cell-independent antigens, including many microbial constituents, are able to stimulate B cells directly or with the help of non-thymus-derived accessory cells. This is particularly true for polysaccharides, which form the capsules of many bacteria, e.g. *Pneumococcus* and *Haemophilus*.

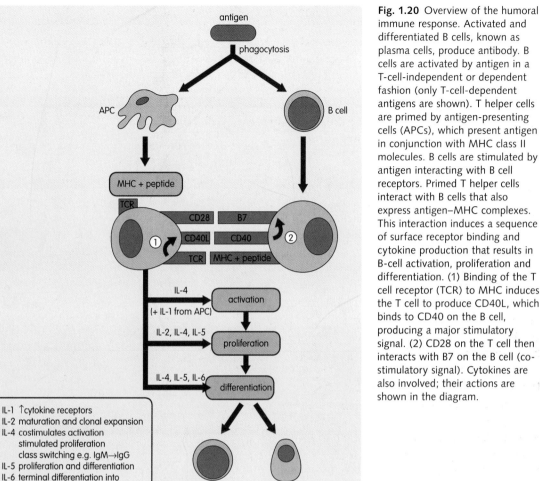

Fig. 1.20 Overview of the humoral immune response. Activated and differentiated B cells, known as plasma cells, produce antibody. B cells are activated by antigen in a T-cell-independent or dependent fashion (only T-cell-dependent antigens are shown). T helper cells are primed by antigen-presenting cells (APCs), which present antigen in conjunction with MHC class II molecules. B cells are stimulated by antigen interacting with B cell receptors. Primed T helper cells interact with B cells that also express antigen–MHC complexes. This interaction induces a sequence of surface receptor binding and cytokine production that results in B-cell activation, proliferation and differentiation. (1) Binding of the T cell receptor (TCR) to MHC induces the T cell to produce CD40L, which binds to CD40 on the B cell, producing a major stimulatory signal. (2) CD28 on the T cell then interacts with B7 on the B cell (co-stimulatory signal). Cytokines are also involved; their actions are shown in the diagram.

Structure and function of antibody

The structure of immunoglobulin is shown in Fig. 1.22. Immunoglobulin molecules (using IgG as an example) are composed of two identical heavy and two identical light chains, linked by disulphide bridges. The light chains consist of one variable and one constant domain, while the heavy chain contains one variable and three constant domains. Digestion of IgG with papain produces two types of fragment:

1. Two Fab fragments (bind antigen) consisting of the light chain and two domains of the heavy chain (denoted VH and CH1)
2. One Fc fragment (binds complement) consisting of the remainder of the heavy chain (CH2 and CH3).

The light chain
The light chain comprises two domains:

- The amino (N) terminal domain is variable and is the site of antigen binding
- The constant domain at the carboxy (C) terminal.

The constant region can be κ or λ, but both light chains within an Ig molecule will be the same; ~60% of human light chains are κ.

The heavy chain
The heavy chain has a variable domain attached to several constant domains. There are five classes of immunoglobulin (Ig) in humans: IgG, IgA, IgM, IgE and IgD. The heavy chain determines the immunoglobulin class. The heavy chain can be γ (IgG), α (IgA), μ (IgM), ε (IgE) or δ (IgD). IgG, IgA and IgD

Fig. 1.21 Clonal selection of B cells. During B cell activation, the antigen-binding region of the immunoglobulin gene undergoes hypermutation. Clonal selection ensures that cells that produce the best antibody are selected and that non-functional or self-reactive B cells are deleted. This process occurs within the germinal centres of lymphoid follicles.

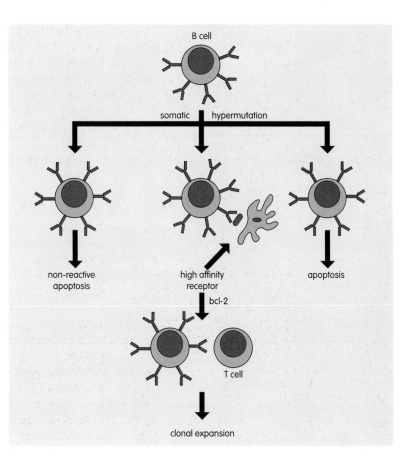

have three constant domains with a hinge region; IgM and IgE have four constant domains but no hinge region.

The variable domain

Each variable domain exhibits three regions that are hypervariable. The hypervariable regions on both light and heavy chains are closely aligned in the immunoglobulin molecule. Together, they form the antigen-binding site and therefore determine the molecule's specificity.

The hinge region

The hinge is a peptide sequence located between the first and second constant domains in the heavy chain. It allows the Fab regions to move against the Fc region from 0 to 90°. This allows greater interaction with epitopes. The hinge region is also the site of the interchain disulphide bonds.

Classes of antibody

The different properties of the immunoglobulin classes are shown in Fig. 1.23. Different Ig classes

and subclasses are specific to each species. IgG, IgE and IgD are monomeric, secreted IgA (sIgA) is usually present as a dimer, and secreted IgM as a pentamer. The sIgA molecule is made up of two IgA monomers: a J chain and a secretory piece. The IgA dimer (J chain) is produced by submucosal plasma cells and enters the mucosal epithelial cell via receptor-mediated endocytosis, binding to the poly-Ig receptor. Having passed from the basal to the luminal surface of the epithelial cell, the IgA dimer is secreted across the mucosa, with part of the poly-Ig receptor (the secretory piece) still attached.

The functions of antibodies

The functions of Igs are shown in Fig. 1.24.

Lymphatic drainage and lymph nodes

Lymph nodes are secondary lymphoid organs. They provide a site for lymphocytes to interact with antigen and other cells of the immune system.

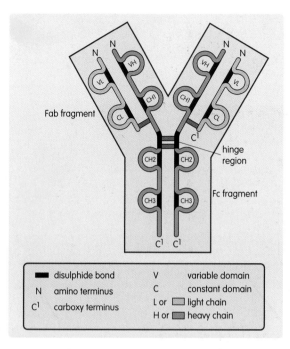

Fig. 1.22 Structure of IgG. Immunoglobulins are composed from two identical light and two identical heavy chains. The chains are divided into domains, each of which is an immunoglobulin fold. The variable domains form the antigen-binding site. Digestion of the immunoglobulin molecule with papain produces an Fc portion (which binds complement) and two Fab portions (which bind antigen).

At the arterial end of capillaries, water and low-molecular-weight solutes leak out into tissue spaces to create interstitial fluid. Most interstitial fluid returns to the venous circulation at the venous end of capillaries (due to pressure gradients). The remainder leaves the interstitial space via the lymphatic system. Once interstitial fluid has entered a lymphatic vessel it is known as lymph. Lymphatic vessels are present in almost all tissues and organs of the body.

Lymphatic circulation

The lymphatic system acts as a passive drainage system to return interstitial fluid to the systemic circulation; lymph is not pumped around the body. Lymph vessels therefore contain numerous valves to prevent backflow of lymph. Afferent lymph vessels carry lymph into lymph nodes. They empty into the subcapsular sinus and lymph percolates through the node. Each node is drained by only one efferent vessel.

Lymph returns to the circulation at lympho-venous junctions. These are located at the junction of the right subclavian vein and right internal jugular vein (which empties the right lymphatic duct) and at the junction of the left subclavian vein and left internal jugular vein (which empties the thoracic duct).

Fig. 1.23 Properties of the five immunoglobulin (Ig) classes

	IgG	IgA	IgM	IgE	IgD
Physical properties					
Molecular weight (kDa)	150	300	900	190	150
Serum concentration (mg/mL)	13.5	3.5	1.5	0.0003	0.03
Number of subunits	1	2	5	1	1
Heavy chain	γ	α	μ	ε	δ
Subclasses	4	2	—	—	—
Biological activities					
Present in secretions	✗	✓	✓	✗	✗
Crosses placenta	✓	✗	✗	✗	✗
Complement fixation	✓	✓	✓✓✓	✗	✗
Binds phagocytic receptors	✓	✗	✓	✗	✗
Binds mast cell receptors	✓	✗	✗	✓	✗
Other features					
Main role	Main circulatory Ig for secondary immune response	Major Ig in secretions	Main Ig in primary immune response	Allergy and antiparasitic response	Expressed on naïve B cell; function not known

Fig. 1.24 Summary of the functions of immunoglobulins

Function	Notes
Opsonization	Phagocytic cells have antibody (Fc) receptors, thus antibody can facilitate phagocytosis of antigen
Agglutination	Antigen and antibody (IgG or IgM) clump together because immunoglobulin can bind more than one epitope simultaneously. IgM is more efficient because it has a high valency (10 antigen-binding sites)
Neutralization	Binding to pathogens or their toxins prevents their attachment to cells
Antibody-dependent cell-mediated cytotoxicity (ADCC)	The antibody–antigen complex can bind to cytotoxic cells (e.g. cytotoxic T cells, NK cells) via the Fc component of the antibody, thus targeting the antigen for destruction
Complement activation	IgG and IgM can activate the classical pathway; IgA can activate the alternative pathway
Mast cell degranulation	Cross-linkage of IgE bound to mast cells and basophils results in degranulation
Protection of the neonate	Transplacental passage of IgG and the secretion of sIgA in breast milk protect the newborn

sIgA, secretory immunoglobulin A; NK, natural killer.

Lymph nodes

Lymph nodes act as filters, 'sampling' lymphatic fluid for bacteria, viruses and foreign particles. APCs, loaded with antigen, also migrate through lymph nodes. They are present throughout the lymphatic system, often occurring at junctions of the lymphatic vessels. Lymph nodes frequently form chains, and may drain a specific organ or area of the body.

Lymph nodes act as sites for initiation of the adaptive immune response. Antigen is sampled, processed and presented by several professional APCs (macrophages and dendritic cells).

Lymphocyte recirculation

Lymphocytes move continuously between blood and lymph. Efferent lymph contains more lymphocytes than afferent lymph because:

- Antigenic challenge results in stimulation and proliferation of lymphocytes
- Lymphocytes enter the lymph node directly from blood.

Lymphocyte recirculation is essential for a normal immune response (Fig. 1.25). Approximately 1–2% of the lymphocytic pool recirculates each hour. This increases the chances of an antigenically committed lymphocyte encountering complementary antigen.

Lymphocytes tend to recirculate to similar tissues. For example, an activated lymphocyte that has migrated from the skin to a local lymph node is most likely to migrate back to the skin following transport in the blood. Similarly, lymphocytes activated in mucosal-associated lymphoid tissue (MALT) will return to MALT. This recirculation is governed by the expression of molecules on both the lymphocyte and surface endothelium. These molecules, called integrins, confer specificity to lymphocyte recirculation. This fine tuning of lymphocyte recirculation is known as lymphocyte homing. Areas of endothelium through which lymphocytes migrate are known as high endothelial venules (HEVs). Lymphocytes activated in MALT express $\alpha_4\beta_7$ integrins that interact with MadCAM-1, an adhesion molecule only expressed on HEVs in MALT.

Lymphadenopathy

Lymph nodes can become enlarged (lymphadenopathy) for several reasons, including infection. Causes of lymphadenopathy are outlined on page 102.

Lymphadenopathy can be a sign of infection. Understanding the drainage of lymph can lead you to the source of infection.

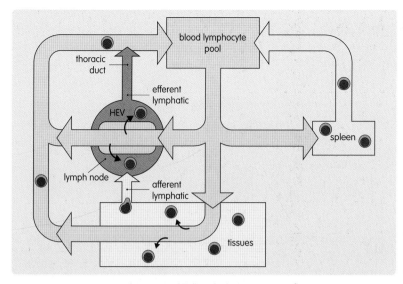

Fig. 1.25 Lymphocyte recirculation. Lymphocytes can enter lymph nodes via specialized high endothelial venules or in lymph. They leave the node in lymph that is returned to the systemic circulation via the right lymphatic duct or thoracic duct. HEV, high endothelial venule.

Mucosal-associated lymphoid tissue (MALT)

MALT consists of unencapsulated subepithelial lymphoid tissue found in the gastrointestinal, respiratory and urogenital tracts (Fig. 1.26). It can be subdivided into:

- Organized lymphoid tissue, e.g. tonsils, appendix, Peyer's patches
- Diffuse lymphoid tissue located in the lamina propria of intestinal villi and lungs.

Organized lymphoid tissue

Respiratory tract
MALT in the nose and bronchi includes the:

- Lingual, palatine and nasopharyngeal tonsils
- Adenoids
- Bronchial nodules.

The respiratory system is exposed to a large number of organisms every day, most of which are cleared by the mucociliary escalator. Microorganisms that are not removed are presented by dendritic cells in the bronchi and stimulate germinating centres.

Gastrointestinal tract
Peyer's patches are organized submucosal lymphoid follicles present throughout the large and small intestine, being particularly prominent in the lower ileum. The structure of a Peyer's patch is shown in Fig. 1.27.

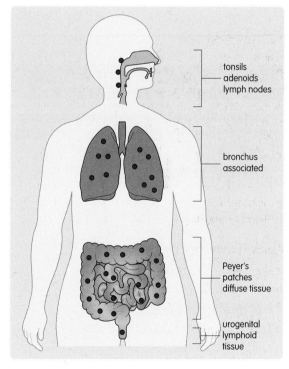

Fig. 1.26 Anatomical location of mucosal-associated lymphoid tissue (MALT). MALT is found in the nasal cavity, throat, respiratory tract, gastrointestinal tract and urogenital tract. Immune cells activated in MALT will home only to other mucosal sites.

Fig. 1.27 Structure of a Peyer's patch. Peyer's patches are found in the gastrointestinal tract. Microbes are transported across specialized epithelial M cells in pinocytotic vesicles into a dome-shaped area. Antigen-presenting cells then process and present antigen to T cells. T helper cells can then activate B cells within the follicle.

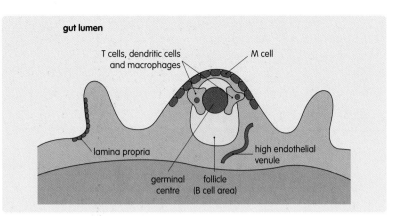

Lymphocyte trafficking in MALT

Mucosal lymphocytes generally recirculate within the mucosal lymphoid system. This occurs through recognition between specific adhesion molecules on the surfaces of lymphocytes from Peyer's patches and corresponding ligands on the venular endothelium.

CELL-MEDIATED IMMUNITY

Cell-mediated immunity is mediated by T lymphocytes, macrophages and NK cells. The cell-mediated immune system is involved in the elimination of:

- Intracellular pathogens and infected cells (mainly viruses, mycobacteria and fungi)
- Tumour cells
- Foreign grafts.

The thymus plays an important role in cell-mediated immunity because it is the site of T cell maturation.

The thymus gland

The thymus is important for the production of T lymphocytes. T lymphocyte differentiation begins in the bone marrow (see p. 67) before early precursor cells migrate to the thymus. In the thymus, immature T lymphocytes undergo random recombination of their T cell receptor genes. Some of the resulting T cell receptors will be specific for pathogens and others for normal self-antigens. The role of the thymus is to select for cells that recognize self-MHC, and negatively select those T cells that recognize self-antigen with self-MHC.

The thymus is a gland with two lobes, located in the anterior part of the superior mediastinum, posterior to the sternum and anterior to the great vessels and upper part of the heart. It can extend superiorly into the roof of the neck and inferiorly into the anterior mediastinum. It receives its blood supply from the inferior thyroid and internal thoracic arteries. Each lobe is surrounded by a capsule and divided into multiple lobules by fibrous septa known as trabeculae. Each lobule is divided into two regions (Fig. 1.28):

- An outer cortex
- An inner medulla.

Immature thymocytes (T cell progenitors) enter the thymus gland via the cortex, where they rapidly proliferate and rearrange their T cell receptor genes. The thymus expresses many of the body's proteins (e.g. insulin) so that T cells which recognize this self-antigen can be forced to undergo apoptosis—so-called negative selection. T cells that are able to bind MHC to some extent will proliferate—positive selection. A much smaller and more mature group of thymocytes survives to enter the medulla. Thymocytes continue to mature in the medulla and eventually leave the thymus, via postcapillary venules, as mature, antigen-specific, immunocompetent T cells. In total, only 1–5% of thymocytes in the thymus reach maturity, the remainder undergoing programmed cell death (apoptosis).

Stromal cells of the thymus

The remainder of the thymic lobule is composed of a network of epithelial cells, known collectively as stromal cells. They interact with developing thymo-

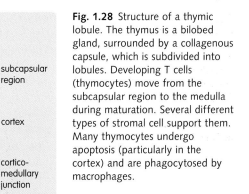

Fig. 1.28 Structure of a thymic lobule. The thymus is a bilobed gland, surrounded by a collagenous capsule, which is subdivided into lobules. Developing T cells (thymocytes) move from the subcapsular region to the medulla during maturation. Several different types of stromal cell support them. Many thymocytes undergo apoptosis (particularly in the cortex) and are phagocytosed by macrophages.

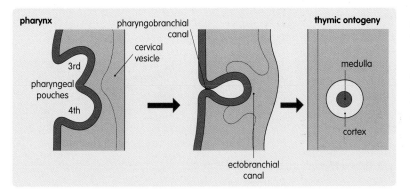

Fig. 1.29 Embryological development of the thymus. The thymus develops from the third (and possibly fourth) pharyngeal pouch. This forms the medulla, which is surrounded by the ectobranchial canal formed from the cervical vesicle. The thymus is developed by 8 weeks of gestation.

cytes and produce several hormones that are essential for their differentiation and maturation.

Embryological origin of the thymus

The human embryonic thymus develops from the third pharyngeal pouch during week 4 or 5 of gestation (Fig. 1.29). The thymus gland is formed by week 8, and is fully differentiated and producing viable lymphocytes by week 17. The third pharyngeal pouch also gives rise to the parathyroid glands. Lymphoid stem cells are produced by the fetal liver and spleen, and by bone marrow from 6 months' gestation.

Thymic hypoplasia

Although it continues to grow until puberty, the relative size of the thymus gland decreases over this period. After puberty there is a real reduction in size and, by adulthood, it is composed largely of adipose tissue and continues to produce far fewer T lympho-

cytes. This means it is harder for adults to recover from immunological damage caused by, for example, HIV or immunosuppressive drugs.

In DiGeorge syndrome, the thymus fails to develop. Consequently, there is an absence of circulating T cells and a reduction in cell-mediated immunity. The mother provides no passive T cell immunity after birth and infants present early with infections.

T lymphocytes
Functions of different T cell phenotypes

The different types of T cell can be differentiated by cell-surface molecules and function. There are two different types of T cell receptor (TCR), which have different functions. T cells expressing αβ-TCRs account for at least 95% of circulatory T cells. They become cytotoxic, helper or suppressor cells and, unless specified otherwise, account for all the T cells mentioned in this book. T cells expressing a γδ-TCR are present at mucosal surfaces and their specificity is biased towards certain bacterial and viral antigens. Some γδ-T cells can recognize antigen independently of an APC. These T cells are usually cytotoxic in their actions. They differ from NK cells because they detect antigen rather than the presence or absence of MHC class I molecules. They are part of the adaptive system, because their action is specific and shows evidence of immunological memory.

T helper cells

T helper (Th) cells play a key role in the development of the immune response:

- They determine the epitopes that are targeted by the immune system via their interactions with antigen in conjunction with class II MHC molecules on APCs
- They determine the nature of the immune response directed against target antigens, e.g. cytotoxic T cell response or antibody response
- They are required for normal B cell function (see p. 4).

Most Th cells are CD4$^+$ and can be divided into four subsets on the basis of the cytokines they secrete:

1. Th0
2. Th1
3. Th2
4. Treg.

Th0 cells arise as a result of initial short-term stimulation of naïve T cells; they are capable of secreting a broad spectrum of cytokines. Prolonged stimulation results in the emergence of Th1 and Th2 subsets. The cytokines released by the Th1 and Th2 subsets modulate one another's secretion. The different cytokine profiles of the Th1 and Th2 subsets reflect their different immunological functions (Fig. 1.30). The fourth type of helper T cell has a regulatory role. If autoreactive T cells manage to escape negative selection in the thymus, they need to be inhibited in the peripheral tissues. Regulatory T cells are capable of preventing this immune response. Their action is unknown but is thought to be via cytokines, including transforming growth factor-β (TNF-β) IL-5, IL-6 and IL-10.

Cytotoxic T cells

Most cytotoxic T (Tc) lymphocytes are CD8$^+$ and recognize antigen in conjunction with class I MHC molecules (endogenous antigen). They lyse target cells via the same mechanisms as NK cells (see p. 67).

Development of T cells

T cell precursors are produced in the bone marrow and are transported to the thymus for development and maturation. The aim of T cell development and maturation is to select T cells with receptors that can recognize foreign antigens in conjunction with self-MHC. Cells with non-functioning receptors or that are strongly self-reactive are destroyed (Fig. 1.31).

Positive selection

Positive selection occurs in the thymic cortex. T cells that are capable of binding self-MHC are allowed to live, i.e. they are positively selected for, and T cells that do not recognize self-MHC die. Furthermore, T cells that interact with MHC class I lose their CD4 (they are now CD8 T cells) and T cells that interact with MHC class II lose their CD8 (becoming CD4 T cells); this is MHC restriction. T cells that do not interact with the MHC molecules undergo

Fig. 1.30 Differences between the T helper 1 (Th1) and T helper 2 (Th2) cell subsets

	Th1 cells	Th2 cells
Cytokines secreted	IL-2, IL-3, IFN-γ, TNF-β	IL-3, IL-4, IL-5, IL-10, IL-13
Functions	• Responsible for classical cell-mediated immunity reactions such as delayed-type hypersensitivity and cytotoxic T cell activation • Involved in responses to intracellular pathogens • Activate macrophages	• Promote B cell activation • Involved in allergic diseases and responses to helminthic infections • Involved in responses to intracellular pathogens

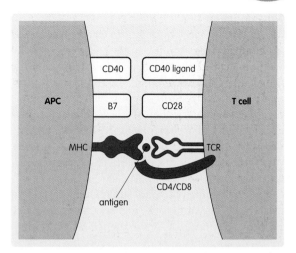

Fig. 1.32 Activation of T cells. Several interactions with antigen-presenting cells (APCs) are required to activate T cells. The T cell receptor (TCR) and CD4 or CD8 bind to MHC and antigen. CD28 on the T cell binds to B7 on the APC, providing a co-stimulatory signal. MHC, major histocompatibility complex.

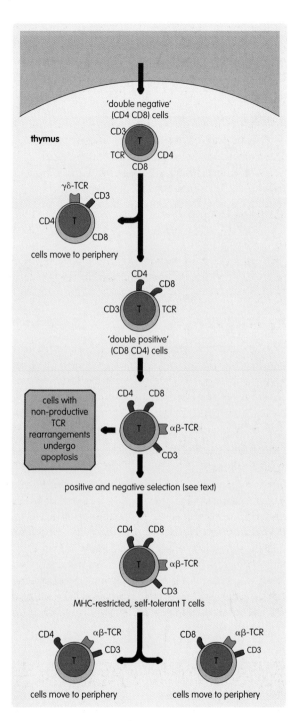

apoptosis, as they do not receive a protective signal as a result of the TCR–MHC interaction.

Negative selection
T cells that are positively selected, but have high affinity for MHC molecules and self-antigen, undergo negative selection.

T cell activation
T cells are activated by interactions between the TCR and peptide bound to MHC. Activation also requires a 'second message' from the antigen-presenting cell. This process is shown in Fig. 1.32. Once T cells are activated they produce a wide range of molecules with several functions. These are primarily cytokines, which may be pro- or anti-inflammatory (see Fig. 1.30) or involved in activation of other immune cells.

Fig. 1.31 Development of T cells in the thymus. Cells entering the thymus to become T cells are negative for CD4, CD8, CD3 and the T cell receptor (TCR). Rearrangement of the genes encoding the TCR will produce three cell lines: (1) CD4$^+$ $\alpha\beta$-TCR; (2) CD8$^+$ $\alpha\beta$-TCR; and (3) CD4$^-$CD8$^-$ $\gamma\delta$-TCR. The β- or γ-chain genes rearrange first. If a functional β-chain is formed, both CD4 and CD8 are upregulated and the α-chain gene rearranges. The resultant T cells are positively selected if their TCR is functional, but negatively selected if they react too strongly. The majority of thymocytes will undergo apoptosis due to positive or negative selection. MHC, major histocompatibility complex.

Superantigens

T cells can be activated in a non-specific fashion by superantigens. Superantigens cross-link between the V-β domain of the TCR and a class II MHC molecule on an antigen-presenting cell. Cross-linking is independent of the peptide binding cleft but depends on the framework region of the V-β domain. This means that one superantigen is able to activate about 5% of T cells, far more than normal antigen. An example of a T cell superantigen is staphylococcal enterotoxin.

Superantigens result in polyclonal activation effectively 'crowding-out' the specific, protective immune response. A consequence of polyclonal activation can be autoimmune disease. Superantigen can also result in the deletion of a large number of T cells by inducing negative selection in the thymus.

Toxic shock syndrome

Toxins produced by staphylococci and streptococci can act as superantigens, producing the clinical picture of 'toxic shock syndrome', where a seemingly innocuous stimulus such as a graze can lead to fever, a diffuse macular rash, hypotension and shock.

RESPONSE TO TISSUE DAMAGE

Inflammation is a non-specific response evoked by tissue injury. The aims of the process are:

- Removal of the causative agent, e.g. microbes or toxins
- Removal of dead tissue
- Replacement of dead tissue with normal tissue, or scar formation.

Inflammation is defined clinically by the presence of redness, swelling and pain, and histologically by the presence of oedema and white cells in a tissue.

Acute inflammation

Acute inflammation is the immediate response to cell injury. It is of short duration (a few hours to a few days) and is triggered by a range of insults, including chemical or thermal damage and infection. Infection is sensed by resident macrophages, through Toll-like receptors, which then release cytokines, attracting neutrophils to the site of infection.

In other instances, inflammation is initiated by resident mast cells, which tend to attract eosinophils. Once inflammation is initiated, several changes occur in vascular endothelium to allow attachment and extravasation of leucocytes—primarily neutrophils but also monocytes and lymphocytes. Attachment and extravasation require the presence of surface molecules on both the endothelium and leucocytes. The acute inflammation process is mediated by many different chemicals.

Vascular changes

Tissue injury results in the release of chemical mediators (cytokines, chemokines and histamine) that act on local blood vessels. The main changes that occur are:

- Vasodilatation: causing increased blood flow and therefore redness and heat
- Slowing of the circulation and increased vascular permeability: formation of an inflammatory exudate results in swelling
- Entry of inflammatory cells, especially neutrophils, into the tissues.

Leucocyte extravasation

Neutrophils adhere to the vessel wall and then pass between the endothelial cells into the tissues. This is a multistep process involving:

31

- Margination: adherence of neutrophils to the vessel wall (Fig. 2.1)
- Diapedesis (extravasation): neutrophils move between endothelial cells into the tissue
- Chemotaxis: due to the release of several chemotactic agents (Fig. 2.2).

Integrin molecules allow immune cells to target specific sites (a process known as homing). To interact successfully with the extracellular matrix, neutrophils must express β_1-integrins, a set of adhesion molecules that can bind to collagen and laminin.

Fig. 2.1 Margination and extravasation (diapedesis) of neutrophils

Margination	Extravasation
Phase I 'Tethering and rolling' Weak interactions between: • L-selectin constitutively expressed on leucocytes • P- and E-selectin that are induced on endothelial cells	Further activator signals result in a conformational change in the leucocyte Metalloproteases are used to detach the cell from the endothelium, before it penetrates the endothelial basement membrane
Phase II 'Activation and strengthening' • Rapid induction of integrins on leucocytes, e.g. CD11b:CD18 (Mac-1) and CD11a:CD18 (LFA-1) on neutrophils • Integrins bind to ICAM molecules expressed constitutively on endothelial cells Phase II is triggered by chemokines	

Neutrophils adhere to vessel walls via cell adhesion molecules (CAMs). CAMs can be members of the immunoglobulin gene superfamily, the selectin family or the integrin family. A variety of inflammatory mediators modifies the expression or alters the affinity of CAMs. Margination is a two-phase process that is followed by cellular migration. ICAM, intercellular adhesion molecule.

Fig. 2.2 Overview of the mediators of acute inflammation

Action	Mediators
Increased vascular permeability	Histamine, bradykinin, C3a, C5a, leukotrienes C_4, D_4, E_4, PAF
Vasodilatation	Histamine, prostaglandins, PAF
Pain	Bradykinin, prostaglandins
Leucocyte adhesion	LTB_4, IL-1, TNF-α, C5a
Leucocyte chemotaxis	C5a, C3a, IL-8, PAF, LTB_4, fibrin and collagen fragments
Acute phase response	IL-1, TNF-α, IL-6
Tissue damage	Proteases and free radicals

IL, interleukin; LT, leukotriene; PAF, platelet-activating factor; TNF, tumour necrosis factor.

Once neutrophils reach a site of inflammation, they phagocytose foreign particles and release enzymes (see Chapter 1). Leucocytes can release proteases and metabolites during chemotaxis and phagocytosis, which are potentially harmful to the host. Neutrophils die during this process, creating pus.

Chemical mediators of inflammation

A variety of chemical mediators are produced during an inflammatory response. They usually have short half-lives and are rapidly inactivated by a variety of systems. A summary of their actions is given in Fig. 2.2.

Cell membrane phospholipid metabolites
Prostaglandins (PGs) and leukotrienes (LTs) are derived from the metabolism of arachidonic acid. Platelet-activating factor (PAF) is also an important mediator.

Cytokines
Cytokines such as IL-8 and IL-1, and tumour necrosis factor-α (TNF-α) act to:

- Induce expression of cell adhesion molecules (CAMs) on the endothelium, thus enhancing leucocyte adhesion
- Attract neutrophils to the area of injury
- Induce prostacyclin (PGI$_2$) production
- Induce PAF synthesis
- Mediate the development of the acute phase response
- Stimulate fibroblast proliferation and increase collagen synthesis.

The complement system
This is discussed in Chapter 1.

The kinin system
Bradykinin is released following activation of the kinin system by Hageman factor (factor XII). Bradykinin increases vascular permeability and mediates pain.

The coagulation system
The coagulation system is activated at sites of vascular injury (see p. 111). Fibrinopeptides produced during coagulation are chemotactic for neutrophils and increase vascular permeability. Thrombin also promotes fibroblast proliferation and leucocyte adhesion.

The fibrinolytic system
Plasmin (see p. 120) has several functions in the inflammatory process, including:

- Activation of complement via C3
- Cleavage of fibrin to form 'fibrin degradation products', which may increase vascular permeability.

Results of acute inflammation

There are several possible outcomes resulting from acute inflammation. These include:

- Regrowth and resolution
- Healing by collagenous scar formation
- Abscess formation
- Chronic inflammation.

Chronic inflammation

Chronic inflammation arises:

- When the causative agent cannot be eliminated and antigenic persistence occurs. This may be due to deficiencies in the host response or certain microorganisms, e.g. *Mycobacterium tuberculosis*, which have evolved to evade the immune response
- As a result of persistent autoimmune reactions, e.g. systemic lupus erythematosus (SLE) and rheumatoid arthritis. The body is, of course, incapable of clearing autoantigens.

The key cells of chronic inflammation are macrophages, lymphocytes and plasma cells. This is in marked contrast to acute inflammation, which is characterized primarily by a neutrophilic inflammation. Ongoing inflammation is associated with tissue destruction, but also healing.

In chronic inflammation, macrophage numbers are increased because they are recruited by chemotactic factors (e.g. platelet-derived growth factor (PDGF) and C5a) and are prevented from leaving by migration inhibition factor. Macrophage secretory products mediate characteristic features of chronic inflammation:

- TNF probably has a key role in maintaining chronic inflammation at a local level. When it is secreted at high levels it has systemic effects, including weight loss (through fat catabolism and appetite inhibition) and fatigue
- Tissue damage via proteases and oxygen radicals

33

Fig. 2.3 Overview of chronic inflammation. Macrophages can be activated by T cells or by non-immune mechanisms. Activated macrophages persist at sites of chronic inflammation because of persistent stimulation. They release a number of molecules, which produce the characteristic features of chronic inflammation. Macrophages act as antigen-presenting cells to T cells, which can then activate further macrophages.

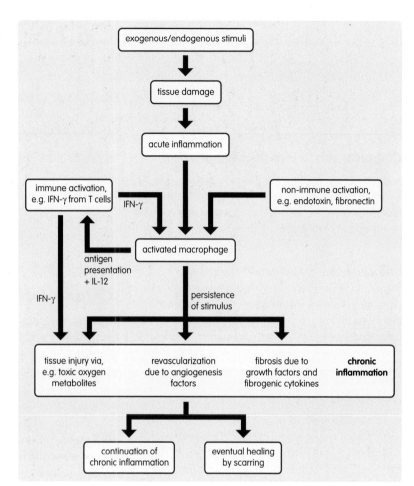

- Revascularization via angiogenic factors
- Fibroblast migration and proliferation via growth factors (e.g. PDGF) and cytokines (IL-2, TNF-α)
- Collagen synthesis via growth factors (e.g. PDGF) and cytokines (IL-1, TNF-α)
- Remodelling via collagenases
- Simulation of T cell activity by secretion of IL-12.

Lymphocytes and plasma cells are also present at the site of inflammation. In the case of chronic infections, both macrophages and T cells are required to control infection. An overview of chronic inflammation is given in Fig. 2.3.

Inflammation in disease

Inflammation is intended to protect the host but can, under certain circumstances, prove destructive.

Antigenic persistence results in the continued activation and accumulation of macrophages. This leads to the formation of epithelioid cells (slightly modified macrophages) and granuloma formation (Fig. 2.4). TNF-α is needed for granuloma formation and maintenance. Interferon-γ (IFN-γ), released by activated T cells, causes macrophage transformation into epithelioid and multinucleate giant cells (which arise from the fusion of several macrophages). The granuloma is surrounded by a cuff of lymphocytes and the migration of fibroblasts results in increased collagen synthesis. Caseous necrotic areas (dry, 'cheese-like' white mass of degenerated tissue) might be present in the centre of a granuloma.

The nature of the damaging stimulus determines the type of granuloma formed. Inert particles (e.g. silica in the lungs) are predominantly surrounded by macrophages. Microorganisms such as *M. tuberculosis* (which causes tuberculosis) induce a persis-

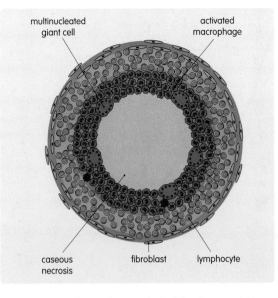

Fig. 2.4 A granuloma, showing typical focal accumulation of lymphocytes and macrophages around a central area of caseous necrosis.

tent, delayed-type hypersensitivity (DTH) response, resulting in granuloma formation in the lung and possibly leading to cavitation (see p. 42). The granuloma formed is characterized by focal accumulation of lymphocytes and macrophages. Phagocytosis of mycobacteria is not usually effective because the microorganism can survive and multiply within macrophages. The granulomatous response, although preventing spread of infection, is harmful to the host.

IMMUNE RESPONSE TO PATHOGENS

Immune response to viral infection

Viruses do not always kill host cells but budding and release of new viral particles often causes the cells to lyse. The immune system can act to prevent infection, or spread of infection, or to eliminate an intracellular target once infection has occurred.

Humoral immunity to viruses

The humoral response is involved in preventing entry to, and viral replication within, cells.

Antibody

Antibodies can bind to free virus and prevent its attachment and entry to a cell; this is referred to as neutralization of virus particles (IgG for hepatitis B and IgA for influenza). Antibodies can also bind to viral proteins expressed on the surface of infected cells. Antibody bound to cells can initiate antibody-dependent cell-mediated cytotoxicity (ADCC) and complement activation, and acts as an opsonin for phagocytes.

Responses directed against free virus are considered to be the most important in vivo, and antibodies are therefore important early in the course of infection to prevent spread of virus between cells.

Interferon

Interferons (IFNs) are produced by virally infected cells. IFN-α and IFN-β act on neighbouring uninfected cells and inhibit transcription and translation of viral proteins. IFN-γ activates macrophages and natural killer (NK) cells and enhances the adaptive immune response by upregulating expression of major histocompatibility complex (MHC) class I and class II molecules.

Cell-mediated immunity to viruses

Cell-mediated mechanisms are important for eliminating virus once infection is established. The cells involved include:

- NK cells: these are cytotoxic for virus-infected cells and participate in ADCC
- Cytotoxic CD8$^+$ T cells: viral peptides are presented on the cell surface in association with class I MHC molecules. CD8$^+$ T cells can destroy these infected cells
- CD4$^+$ T cells: T helper cells are required for the generation of antibody and cytotoxic T cell responses, and the recruitment and activation of macrophages (Th1 help).

An overview of the immune response to viruses is given in Fig. 2.5.

Examples of viral infection and strategies to avoid immunity

Viral infections are common and most are self-limiting. Some, particularly those that can evade the immune response, can be chronic and are potentially fatal (e.g. HIV [see p. 55] and hepatitis B). Different viruses use different strategies to evade the host's immune response:

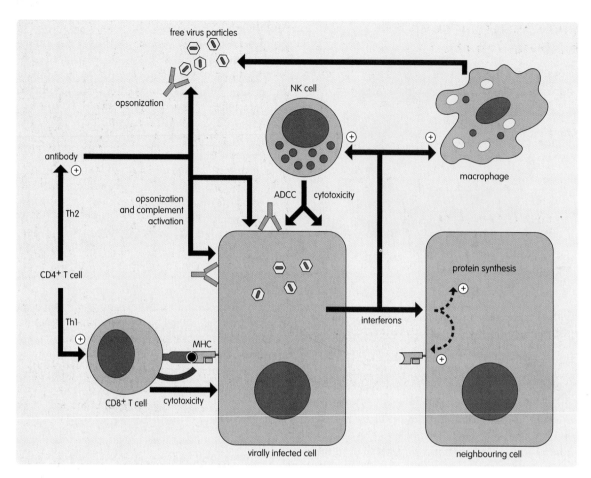

Fig. 2.5 The immune response to viruses. Interferons, produced by virally infected cells, have three important actions. Interferon-α and interferon-β induce an antiviral state in neighbouring cells (inhibition of viral transcription and translation). Interferon-γ activates macrophages and natural killer (NK) cells and upregulates major histocompatibility (MHC) molecules. NK cells kill virally infected cells either by detecting the absence of MHC class I molecules or by antibody-dependent cell-mediated cytotoxicity (ADCC). Macrophages phagocytose opsonized free virus and cell fragments, and produce further interferon. CD8$^+$ (cytotoxic) T cells sense viral peptides presented by MHC class I molecules and destroy the cell. CD4$^+$ (helper) T cells help to activate macrophages and are involved in the generation of antibody and cytotoxic T cell responses.

- Antigenic shift and drift: these are mechanisms of antigenic variation, e.g. influenza
- Polymorphism: e.g. adenovirus, rhinovirus
- Latent virus: e.g. herpes simplex virus (HSV), varicella zoster
- Modulation of MHC expression: cytomegalovirus (CMV), adenovirus, Epstein–Barr virus (EBV), HSV, HIV
- Infection of lymphocytes, e.g. HIV, measles, CMV, EBV.

Antigenic variation, either by mutation or polymorphism, circumvents immunological memory because the virus expresses different immunological targets over time. By becoming latent, virus 'hides' from the immune system. Latent virus often reactivates when the immune system is compromised, suggesting that there must be some interaction between the immune system and the virus even when it is latent. Mechanisms that prevent normal effector functions from being carried out primarily involve downregulation of MHC class I expression. However, viruses can also interfere with IFN or produce inhibitory cytokines. Infection of lymphocytes, and their death, reduces the ability of the immune system to combat viral infection.

Immune response to bacterial infection

Bacteria are prokaryotic organisms. Their cell membrane is surrounded by a peptidoglycan cell wall. Many bacteria also have a capsule of large, branched polysaccharides. Bacteria attach to cells via surface pili, but only some bacteria enter host cells. Different immune mechanisms operate, depending on whether the bacteria are extracellular or intracellular.

Extracellular bacteria

Humoral immunity to extracellular bacteria

Complement

Bacteria activate complement via the lectin or alternative pathways. Activated complement products play a role in the elimination of bacteria, especially C3b (an opsonin), C3a and C5a (anaphylatoxins that recruit leucocytes), and the membrane attack complex (MAC), which can perforate the outer lipid bilayer of Gram-negative bacteria.

Lysozyme

Lysozyme is a naturally occurring antibacterial that attacks N-acetyl muramic acid–N-acetyl glucosamine links in the bacterial cell wall. This results in bacterial lysis.

Antibody

This is the principal defence against extracellular bacteria:

- sIgA binds to bacteria and prevents their binding to epithelial cells; if this response is sufficient, sIgA can prevent the pathogen from entering the body
- Antibody neutralizes bacterial toxins
- Antibody activates complement
- Antibody acts as an opsonin.

Cell-mediated immunity to extracellular bacteria

Phagocytic cells kill most bacteria; C3b and antibody enhance phagocytosis. Bacterial antigens are processed and presented in conjunction with class II MHC to CD4$^+$ T cells. CD4$^+$ T cell help is required for the generation of the antibody response (Th2 help). Cells that present antigen in association with class II MHC include macrophages, dendritic cells

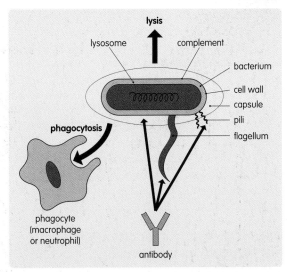

Fig. 2.6 The immune response to extracellular bacteria. The first line of host defence against bacteria is lysozyme. This 'natural antibiotic' attacks N-acetyl muramic acid–N-acetyl glucosamine links in the bacterial cell wall. This, together with complement, leads to bacterial lysis. Antibody is produced against flagella (immobilizing) and pili (prevents attachment). Capsular polysaccharides can induce T-cell-independent antibody. Antibodies aid complement activation and phagocytosis of bacteria.

and B lymphocytes; collectively, these are called professional antigen-presenting cells (APCs). Toll-like receptors on the surface of APCs recognize pathogenic molecules and further potentiate the immune response.

An overview of the immune response to extracellular bacteria is given in Fig. 2.6.

Intracellular bacteria

Humoral immunity to intracellular bacteria

The humoral mechanisms that are employed against extracellular bacteria will be used to try to prevent bacteria causing intracellular infection. However, they will not be effective once the infection is intracellular.

Cell-mediated immunity to intracellular bacteria

Cell-mediated immunity is very important in the defence against intracellular bacterial infections, such as those caused by *M. tuberculosis*:

- Macrophages attempt to phagocytose the bacteria. If the organisms persist, chronic inflammation will ensue. This can lead to delayed (type IV) hypersensitivity (see p. 42)
- Cells infected with bacteria can activate NK cells, which cause cytotoxicity and can activate macrophages
- CD4$^+$ T cells release cytokines that activate macrophages (Th1 help)
- CD8$^+$ T cells recognize antigens presented in conjunction with class I MHC molecules on the surface of infected cells and lyse these cells.

Examples of infection and bacterial strategies to avoid immunity

Bacterial strategies to avoid the immune response must allow one of the following:

- Prevent phagocytosis
- Allow survival within phagocytes
- Prevent complement activation
- Avoid recognition by the immune system.

Strategies to avoid immunity include:

- Capsules can inhibit phagocytosis, e.g. *Streptococcus pneumoniae*, *Haemophilus* spp.
- Killing of phagocytes by toxins, e.g. *Staphylococcus* spp.
- Neutralization of opsonizing IgG, e.g. *Staphylococcus* spp.
- Survival within phagocytes, e.g. *M. tuberculosis*, *Mycobacterium leprae*, *Toxoplasma* spp.
- Inhibition of complement activation, e.g. *Staphylococcus* spp., *Streptococcus* spp., *Haemophilus* spp., *Pseudomonas* spp.
- Polymorphism, e.g. *Streptococcus pneumoniae*, *Salmonella typhi*.

Like viruses, bacteria can be highly polymorphic. Bacteria of the same species can appear to be entirely different to the immune system.

Immune response to protozoal infection

Protozoa are microscopic, single-celled organisms. Fewer than 20 types of protozoa infect humans, although malaria, trypanosomes and *Leishmania* cause significant morbidity and mortality. Protozoa cause intracellular infection, have marked antigenic variation and are often immunosuppressive. They have complex lifecycles, with several different stages, and therefore present the immune system with a variety of challenges. Protozoal infection is often chronic, as the immune system is not very efficient at dealing with these organisms. Most of the pathology of protozoal disease is caused by the immune response.

Humoral immunity against protozoa

Complement and antibody are important during the extracellular stage of infection. This opsonizes the protozoa and can cause lysis or prevent infection.

Cell-mediated immunity against protozoa

- *Phagocytosis* by macrophages, monocytes and neutrophils is an important part of the immune response against protozoa
- *CD4$^+$ T cells* are activated in response to protozoal infection. The subset of CD4$^+$ T cells activated is thought to determine whether the immune response is protective or not. T helper 1 cytokines, e.g. IL-2, IFN-γ, TNF-β, are considered protective
- *Cytotoxic CD8$^+$ T cells* are important in destroying protozoa that replicate within cells, e.g. the sporozoite stage of *Plasmodium falciparum* (which causes malaria)
- *NK cells and mast cells* are often activated in protozoal infection.

Examples of protozoal infection and evasion of the immune response

Protozoa have good mechanisms to prevent the initiation of an immune response. Strategies include:

- Escape into the cytoplasm following phagocytosis, e.g. *Trypanosoma cruzi*
- Prevention of complement actions, e.g. *Leishmania* spp.
- Gene switching to create antigen variation, e.g. trypanosomes
- Immunosuppression, e.g. trypanosomes.

Immune response to worms

Multicellular parasites and worms pose a different problem to the immune system, as they are too large to be phagocytosed by macrophages and neutrophils. These worms tend to live on mucosal surfaces, and the immune system tries to dispose of these parasites by facilitating their expulsion. The immune system does this by secreting toxic chemicals onto mucosal surfaces, stimulating an increase in mucus secretion and smooth muscle contraction, which together result in expulsion of the worm.

Mast cells are stationed in tissues and have a similar sentinel purpose, with respect to worm infection, as that performed by macrophages for other types of infection. Mast cells contain pre-formed granules and, when they recognize parasitic infection through cross-linkage of IgE or possibly Toll-like receptors, they degranulate, releasing their preformed granules and other rapidly synthesized chemicals onto the parasite. They also release proinflammatory cytokines that recruit eosinophils and basophils.

Mast cell preformed granules contain:

- Histamine: causes smooth muscle in the walls of the gut to contract (expel the worm) and smooth muscle of blood vessels to relax
- Proteolytic enzymes: activate the complement system including anaphylatoxins.

The rapidly synthesized chemicals include prostaglandins and leukotrienes, both of which cause vasodilatation and contraction of smooth muscle in gut and bronchial walls.

Eosinophils secrete chemicals similar to those secreted by mast cells, excluding histamine. In addition they secrete:

- Peroxidase that generates hypochlorous acid
- A cationic protein which damages the worm's outer layers and paralyses its nervous system
- A basic protein that also attacks the outer layers of the worm.

Mast cells can be activated by IgE and, although this probably evolved to deal with worm infections, it mediates allergy (type I hypersensitivity).

A note on prion infection

Prions are an abnormal form of a normal host protein. This aberrant protein is able to convert normal protein to the abnormal form; the immune response to prions remains largely unknown.

The most important prion infection in humans is variant Creutzfeldt–Jakob disease (vCJD).

The clinical features of prion infection are:

- Progressive degenerative neurological disease

- Long incubation period—up to 40 years
- Rapid onset to death once symptoms arise.

HYPERSENSITIVITY

Concepts of hypersensitivity

Hypersensitivity is where there is an excessive and therefore inappropriate inflammatory response to any antigen. This inflammatory response results in tissue damage.

Hypersensitivity reactions are normal immunological processes that occur at the wrong time, meaning that each mechanism does have a beneficial purpose when reacting to the correct antigen.

Hypersensitivity can occur in response to:

- An infection that cannot be cleared, e.g. tuberculosis
- A normally harmless exogenous substance, e.g. pollen
- An autoantigen, e.g. DNA in SLE.

Hypersensitivity reactions have been classified, by Gell and Coombs, into four types: I, II, III and IV. Types I, II and III are antibody-mediated; type IV is cell-mediated.

Type I hypersensitivity (immediate hypersensitivity, allergy)

Type I hypersensitivity is mediated by IgE, with resultant and immediate degranulation of mast cells and basophils.

Overproduction of IgE in response to an innocuous environmental antigen occurs in allergy. Individuals with a greater inherited tendency towards type I hypersensitivity reactions are said to be atopic.

Type I hypersensitivity reactions require an initial antigen exposure in order to sensitize the immune system. When atopic individuals are exposed to an allergen they produce lots of IgE specific for that antigen. Mast cells have membrane receptors specific for the Fc portion of IgE, so that mast cells become coated in IgE. The immune system in now said to be sensitized to the allergen. Subsequent exposure to the same antigen, cross-linking mast cell surface IgE, results in release of preformed mediators of inflammation (degranulation). Short-lived basophils with IgE receptors are recruited and also degranulate in response to the antigen.

Mast cells and basophils release their contents within minutes of exposure to an allergen; this is the early phase response. The late phase response, mediated by eosinophils, responds to the same stimulus. This delay occurs as eosinophils have to be mobilized from the bone marrow. Clinically this can manifest itself as a further deterioration in symptoms several hours after initial exposure.

The immune mechanisms of type I reactions are illustrated in Fig. 2.7. Examples of type I reactions include:

- Allergic rhinitis (hay fever): pollens
- Allergic asthma: house-dust mite
- Systemic anaphylaxis: penicillin, peanuts or insect venom.

Atopy is a genetic predisposition to produce IgE in response to many common, naturally occurring allergens. It has a prevalence of 10–30%. Atopic patients can suffer from multiple allergies. The genetic basis of atopy is not known.

When diagnosing type I hypersensitivity, the most important source of information is the history and the timing of events as the effects of allergy occur rapidly—within minutes. Allergy can result in a wide spectrum of symptoms, the most severe being anaphylaxis. This occurs as a consequence of increased vascular permeability and dilatation, causing large amounts of fluid to move out of the circulation and into tissues, leading to a rapid fall in blood pressure. Allergy most often produces symptoms local to the site of allergen entry:

- Skin: results in an urticarial rash or eczema
- Nasal mucosa: results in rhinitis, e.g. hay fever
- Lungs: can result in asthma.

For an allergic reaction to occur, IgE against that specific allergen needs to be present. This can be tested for using skin prick testing (this is not advisable for severe allergy) where a small amount of the suspected allergen is inoculated into the skin together with a positive and a negative control. A positive reaction will result in an itchy red lesion with a weal at the centre; the reaction is strongest after 15–20 minutes, indicating that the patient produces IgE to the tested allergen. Although serum IgE can be directly measured using a blood test, it must be remembered that many people have IgE to some allergens.

Type II hypersensitivity

Type II (or antibody-mediated) hypersensitivity occurs when antibody specific for cell surface antigens is produced. Cell destruction can then result via:

- Complement activation
- Antibody-dependent cell-mediated cytotoxicity (ADCC)
- Phagocytosis.

The immune mechanisms of type II hypersensitivity reactions are summarized in Fig. 2.8.

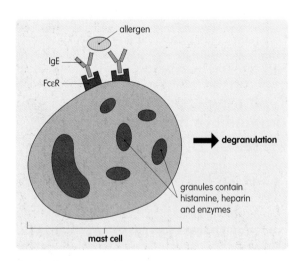

Fig. 2.7 The immune mechanisms of type I hypersensitivity reactions. Cross-linkage of IgE bound to cell surface receptors on mast cells and basophils results in degranulation.

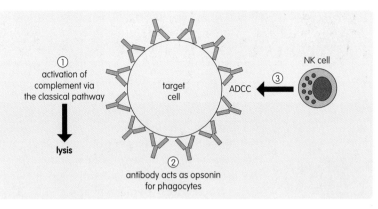

Fig. 2.8 The immune mechanisms of type II hypersensitivity reactions. Antibody bound to cells (either antibody to foreign cells or autoantibody) results in cell death via (1) complement, (2) phagocytes or (3) natural killer (NK) cells. ADCC, antibody-dependent cell-mediated cytotoxicity.

Examples of type II reactions in which complement is activated and cells destroyed are:

- Incompatible blood transfusions
- Haemolytic disease of the newborn
- Autoimmune haemolytic anaemias.

Several diseases are caused by antibody directed against cell surface receptors, which can stimulate or block the receptor. In Graves' disease, stimulating antibodies are directed against the receptor for thyroid stimulating hormone. In myasthenia gravis, antibodies are directed against the acetylcholine receptor. They can destroy the receptor or cause lysis due to complement activation.

Type III hypersensitivity (immune complex)

Antibodies react to soluble antigen by forming lattices of antibody and antigen, called an immune complex. This is a physiological response and is useful, for example, in the removal of bacterial exotoxin. The immune complexes are broken up by complement and transported to the spleen by red blood cells (RBCs) where they are phagocytosed. If there is a rapid influx in antigen that overwhelms these coping strategies, then a type III hypersensitivity reaction occurs (Fig. 2.9). Type III hypersensitivity can occur locally or systemically.

Examples of local type III hypersensitivity include:

- Arthus reaction: intradermal or subcutaneous injection of antigen into a recipient with high levels of appropriate circulating antibody produces localized immune complexes that activate complement and generate acute inflammation

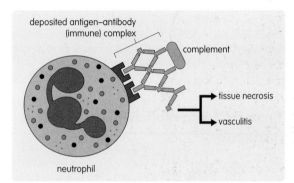

Fig. 2.9 The immune mechanisms of type III hypersensitivity reactions. Immune complexes that are normally removed by phagocytes are deposited in blood vessels or the tissues resulting in severe damage via complement and neutrophils.

- Farmer's lung: inhalation of mould spores
- Pigeon fancier's disease: repeated inhalation of dried pigeon faeces.

Systemic type III hypersensitivity reactions occur when there is a large amount of antibody present throughout the body; this can occur when antigens such as antibiotics are injected into the circulation, or if the antigen is a self-antigen (an autoimmune reaction) such as occurs in SLE.

SLE

Glomerular and synovial cells both contain the receptor CR1, i.e. the receptor on RBCs that picks up the immune complex to take to the spleen. As a result, generalized type III hypersensitivity reactions such as those that occur in SLE are associated with kidney and joint pathology.

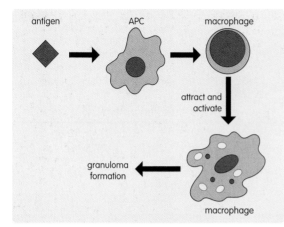

Fig. 2.10 The immune mechanisms of type IV hypersensitivity reactions. These reactions take several days to be initiated because antigen is first presented to T cells, which can then activate macrophages. APC, antigen-presenting cell.

Type IV hypersensitivity (delayed)

Upon first contact with antigen, a subset of CD4+ T helper (Th) cells is activated and clonally expanded (this takes 1–2 weeks). Upon subsequent encounter with the same antigen, sensitized Th cells secrete cytokines. These attract and activate macrophages, which account for more than 95% of the cells involved. Activated macrophages have increased phagocytic ability and can destroy pathogens more effectively. The type IV reaction peaks at 48–72 hours after contact with the antigen (time taken for the recruitment and activation of the macrophages) and is therefore known as delayed-type hypersensitivity. An overview of the immune mechanisms involved is given in Fig. 2.10.

Type IV reactions are important for the clearance of intracellular pathogens. However, if antigen persists, the response can be detrimental to the individual, as the lytic products of the activated macrophages can damage healthy tissues. Examples of antigens that induce a type IV response are:

- Contact antigens such as nickel
- Intracellular pathogens such as *M. tuberculosis*.

Skin testing is performed to detect type IV reactions. Patch testing is used to diagnose antigens causing delayed hypersensitivity in contact dermatitis. The sensitizing antigen is placed on the skin, the area is dressed and left for 48–72 hours. In contrast, when testing for immediate hypersensitivity, a reaction should occur very quickly and skin prick tests are read at 15 minutes after exposure. The tuberculin skin test can be used to determine whether a person has been exposed to *M. tuberculosis*. An intradermal injection of purified protein derivative (PPD) is given to the individual. Previous exposure to *M. tuberculosis* or bacille Calmette–Guérin (BCG) vaccination results in a positive response. This is apparent as a firm, red (due to the intense infiltration of macrophages) lesion at the injection site 48–72 hours after the injection. The skin lesions in both contact dermatitis and tuberculin testing are composed of macrophages and T cells.

ANTI-INFLAMMATORY DRUGS

Anti-inflammatory drugs are used commonly for the treatment of a variety of hypersensitivity reactions. Different types of anti-inflammatory drug are available, including:

- Corticosteroids
- Non-steroidal anti-inflammatory drugs
- Other anti-inflammatory agents.

Corticosteroids

The adrenal cortex releases several steroid hormones into the circulation. Glucocorticoids affect not only carbohydrate and protein metabolism, but also have effects on the immune system, acting as immunosuppressive and anti-inflammatory agents. Several glucocorticoids are available therapeutically, including:

- Hydrocortisone: can be given intravenously in status asthmaticus or topically for inflammatory skin conditions
- Prednisolone: oral preparations are given in many inflammatory or allergic conditions
- Beclometasone: used as an aerosol in asthma or topically for eczema.

Conditions commonly treated with steroids include:

- Inflammatory bowel disease
- Allergic conditions, e.g. asthma
- Severe inflammatory skin conditions
- Severe inflammatory rheumatological conditions.

Corticosteroids work primarily on phagocytes. They inhibit the production of mediators of inflammation (prostaglandins, cytokines) and prevent antigen presentation. At high doses they have direct effects on lymphocytes.

Adverse effects and contraindications

Glucocorticoids cause many adverse effects at the high doses required to produce an anti-inflammatory effect. The clinical features are similar to those seen in Cushing's syndrome and the adverse effects are shown in Fig. 2.11. Steroids are contraindicated if there is evidence of systemic infection. Long-term high dose steroid therapy is usually avoided. When they are used long term, there should be regular checks on blood pressure, blood sugar and bone density.

Non-steroidal anti-inflammatory drugs (NSAIDs)

NSAIDs include a large number of drugs that can be bought over the counter, e.g. aspirin, ibuprofen, diclofenac. They are chemically diverse but all act to inhibit cyclo-oxygenase (Fig. 2.12). This attenuates, but does not abolish, inflammation. As well as their anti-inflammatory effects, NSAIDs have analgesic and antipyretic actions. They are used primarily in conditions where pain is accompanied by inflammation, such as rheumatoid arthritis.

Cyclo-oxygenase (COX) occurs as two isoenzymes: COX1 and COX2. There are advantages to selectively blocking each of the COX enzymes in different circumstances. Selective COX2 inhibitors have reduced gastrointestinal side-effects, as the production of protective prostaglandins in the gastric mucosa is mediated by COX1. Selective COX1 inhibition reduces platelet aggregation, but renders the individual susceptible to gastric inflammation.

Aspirin

Acetylsalicylic acid (aspirin) is anti-inflammatory but causes a lot of adverse effects. As a consequence of this, newer NSAIDs (e.g. ibuprofen) are usually preferred for treatment of inflammatory conditions, because they exhibit fewer side-effects. Aspirin is far

Fig. 2.11 The adverse effects of glucocorticoids

Body system	Symptoms
Gastrointestinal	Dyspepsia, nausea, peptic ulceration, abdominal distension, acute pancreatitis, oesophageal ulceration, candidiasis
Musculoskeletal	Osteoporosis, proximal myopathy, avascular osteonecrosis
Endocrine	Adrenal suppression, menstrual irregularities, hirsutism, weight gain, negative nitrogen and calcium balance, increased appetite, increased susceptibility to infection, diabetes
Neuropsychiatric	Euphoria, psychological dependence, depression, insomnia, aggravation of epilepsy, psychosis
Ophthalmic	Glaucoma, papilloedema, cataracts
Skin	Impaired wound healing, atrophy, easy bruising, striae, telangiectasia, acne

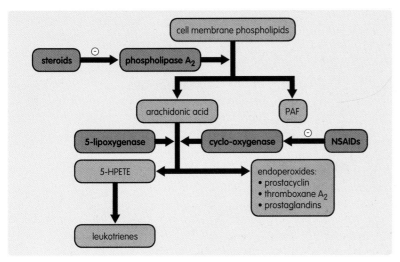

Fig. 2.12 The actions of non-steroidal anti-inflammatory drugs (NSAIDs) in arachidonic acid metabolism. PAF, platelet-activating factor.

more efficient at inhibiting COX1 (hence the side-effects) and is used prophylactically in low doses in people who have had strokes or have ischaemic heart disease because of its ability to inhibit platelet function.

Paracetamol

Paracetamol has good analgesic properties but little effect on inflammation. Thus it is not strictly an NSAID but is usually grouped with them for ease.

Adverse effects and contraindications

Adverse effects with NSAIDs are common. They often cause damage to the mucosa of the gastrointestinal tract because they remove the cytoprotective effects of prostaglandins in the gut; the mucosa becomes ulcerated because of the damaging effects of stomach acid. Many NSAID preparations, e.g. enteric-coating, are designed to reduce ulceration. NSAIDs can also be nephrotoxic and cause bronchospasm. Side-effects of aspirin include nausea, vomiting, epigastric pain and tinnitus.

Other anti-inflammatory drugs

Other anti-inflammatory drugs reduce inflammation via different mechanisms. These include:

- Immunosuppressive drugs, such as ciclosporin and azathioprine (main effects on T cells)
- Methotrexate (main effects on macrophages).

Such drugs are often used in chronic inflammatory conditions, e.g. rheumatoid arthritis, to reduce the need for steroids. Each drug has specific adverse effects and contraindications. Newer approaches use biological agents to block the effects of proinflammatory cytokines. For example, the effects of TNF can be blocked by infliximab (monoclonal anti-TNF) or etanercept (soluble TNF receptor). Both drugs are very effective in the treatment of rheumatoid arthritis and Crohn's disease. However, they can increase the risk of infections, such as tuberculosis, in which TNF normally has a protective role.

INVESTIGATION OF IMMUNE FUNCTION

Electrophoresis

Electrophoresis uses an electric field to separate proteins or nucleic acids on the basis of size, electric charge and other physical properties. An electric current is passed across a support matrix (e.g. cellulose acetate, polyacrylamide gel) or a solution. As particles travel at different rates (because of their different electrical charge and size), they gradually separate to form bands, which can be visualized by staining. Electrophoresis is commonly used to detect excess monoclonal immunoglobulin production in multiple myeloma (see p. 107).

Immunoassays

This is a technique that uses antibody to identify antigen or biological molecules.

ELISA

Enzyme-linked immunosorbent assay (ELISA) is a sensitive test that allows quantitative analysis of the amount of a specific antigen or antigen/antibody complex in a sample.

In an ELISA an enzyme is attached to the antigen under study, and catalyses the conversion of a colourless substrate to a coloured product. The amount of coloured end product is proportional to the amount of antigen and can be measured using a spectrometer.

ELISAs are commonly used to measure specific antibody in a patient's serum so I will use this as a working example.

- A plate containing the antigen for the antibody being tested is exposed to the patient's serum; any of the appropriate antibody present in the serum will bind the antigen on the plate
- The enzyme used to catalyse the production of the coloured product (which is covalently attached to an antibody that is specific for the Fc portion of the antibody in the patient's serum) is added (see Fig. 2.13)
- The enzyme substrate is then added and the colour conversion occurs.

Each of these steps is incubated for a consistent period of time with any excess being washed before the next substance is added.

In addition to the ELISA test we can detect antibody by agglutination, for example:

- Coombs test
- Rheumatoid factor.

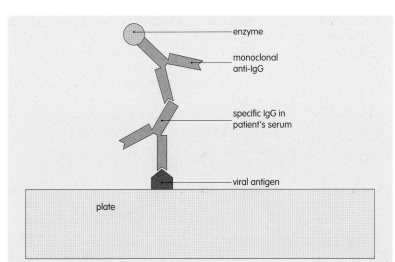

Fig. 2.13 Enzyme-linked immunosorbent assay (ELISA). ELISA can be used to detect antigens but is most commonly used to measure antibody to specific antigen (e.g. a virus) and this is shown. Viral antigen is bound to a plate and the patient's serum added. If specific IgG is present it will bind to the antigen. Enzyme labelled anti-IgG is added (binding to the patient's IgG). The enzyme converts a colourless substrate into a coloured product. The intensity of colour is relative to the amount of antigen.

Flow cytometry and immunofluorescence

Flow cytometry is a useful tool for differentiating between different populations of cells, as well as for counting the number of cells within a sample. This is done by producing a very fine stream of cells in suspension, where only one cell at a time passes through a beam of laser light. Sensors detect when a cell blocks the beam of light and the amount of light scatter identifies the size and granularity of the cell. Various surface antigens on the cell can be bound by monoclonal antibodies (specific for one antigen). The monoclonal antibodies are labelled with dyes that fluoresce under laser light (immunofluorescence). Different types of dye allow the detection of specific antigens (most machines use red and green fluorescence, but up to five colours are used by some machines); CD4 counts (T cell counts) are done in this way.

Measuring cytokines

Cytokines are occasionally measured directly in blood samples. For example, high levels of TNF and IL-6 are seen in septic shock.

Blood samples can also be incubated with antigens and the resultant cytokines measured. For example, if blood incubated with mycobacterial antigen produces IFN-γ, this may indicate exposure to tuberculosis.

Tests for autoimmunity

The presence of autoantibodies can be detected in many rheumatic and endocrine disorders. Rheumatoid factor (RF), commonly seen in rheumatoid arthritis (see p. 49), is an anti-IgG antibody. However, RF is not always present in rheumatoid arthritis and can occur in other rheumatic conditions. It can be detected by agglutination of latex particles or sheep red blood cells that have been coated with immunoglobulin.

Indirect immunofluorescence of a range of tissues can be used to detect autoantibodies to nuclear and cytoplasmic antigens. Specific antibodies, e.g. anti-double-stranded DNA in SLE (for other examples, see Figs 2.17 and 2.18), can be detected by ELISA.

Tests for allergy

See hypersensitivity (p. 39).

ALLERGY

Allergy is due to hypersensitivity reactions to exogenous antigens (known as allergens), mediated by IgE. Allergic symptoms usually result from degranulation of mast cells. This process is mediated by the cross-linking of IgE by allergen. Allergic conditions are therefore type I hypersensitivity reactions. Other types of hypersensitivity cause chronic disease but are not termed allergies. The symptoms of different allergies affect different tissues and can be local or generalized.

Asthma

Asthma is a chronic inflammatory disorder of the airways, characterized by reversible airflow obstruction. The airways become hyper-responsive and exaggerated bronchoconstriction follows a wide variety of stimuli, e.g. exercise or cold air. The symptoms of asthma are cough, wheeze, chest tightness and shortness of breath. Asthma is a common disease and is diagnosed in 5–10% of children. The incidence has risen over the last few decades, particularly in more economically developed countries.

Pollens, house-dust mite faeces and animal fur are the most common allergens. These cause inflammation of the bronchial wall involving:

- Infiltration by eosinophils, mast cells, lymphocytes and neutrophils
- Oedema of the submucosa
- Smooth muscle hypertrophy and hyperplasia
- Thickening of the basement membrane
- Mucous plugging
- Epithelial desquamation.

Asthma is diagnosed by a reversal in airway obstruction (measured by peak expiratory flow rate,

or 'peak flow') of ≥15%, either spontaneously or following the administration of an inhaled β_2-adrenoreceptor agonist (such as salbutamol). This treatment is used for the short-term improvement of symptoms, although inhaled steroids and other immunosuppressive/anti-inflammatory drugs are used prophylactically to prevent asthma attacks.

Atopic/allergic eczema

Eczema or dermatitis can be caused by an allergic response. Dermatitis means skin inflammation. There are several types of dermatitis, including allergic (atopic) eczema (type I hypersensitivity reaction) and contact dermatitis (a type IV hypersensitivity reaction). Contact dermatitis can be diagnosed by patch testing and treatment is primarily by avoidance of the antigen (e.g. nickel).

Atopic eczema is most commonly the result of exposure to pollen or house-dust mite faeces. Common allergens are shown in Fig. 2.14. About 10% of children are diagnosed with eczema. Eczema commonly affects the flexural creases and the fronts of the wrist and ankles. In infancy and adulthood the face and trunk are often involved. The skin lesions are itchy, red, sometimes vesicular and might be dry. Because of itching, the skin is often excoriated, which can lead to lichenification (thickening of the skin). Eczema is often compli-

Fig. 2.14 Summary of allergic reactions

Allergic condition	Common allergens	Features
Systemic anaphylaxis	Drugs Serum Venoms Peanuts	Oedema with increased vascular permeability Leads to tracheal occlusion, circulatory collapse and possibly death
Allergic rhinitis	Pollen (hay fever) Dust-mite faeces (perennial rhinitis)	Sneezing, oedema and irritation of nasal mucosa
Asthma	Pollen Dust-mite faeces	Bronchial constriction, increased mucus production, airway inflammation
Food	Shellfish Milk Eggs Fish Wheat	Itching urticaria and potentially anaphylaxis
Atopic eczema	Pollen Dust-mite faeces Some foods	Itchy inflammation of the skin

cated by superinfection with bacteria, particularly *Staphylococcus aureus*.

The diagnosis of atopic eczema is usually clinical. Total serum IgE, RAST for specific IgE and skin prick testing with common allergens are occasionally performed to confirm the diagnosis of atopic eczema. Treatment of eczema is mainly topical, except in more severe cases, when systemic steroids and immunosuppressants are used. Therapies include:

- Emollients: moisturizes dry skin and reduces itching
- Topical steroids: anti-inflammatory
- Topical antibiotics or antiseptics: in infected eczema
- Oral antihistamine: reduces itching
- Ciclosporin: resistant cases might require immunosuppression.

Skin prick testing

A skin prick test is a useful way of assessing whether a person has IgE to different allergens (see photograph). The response should always be compared to a histamine control. Results should be interpreted carefully as people can have IgE to an allergen without having any symptoms. Conversely, they may show no reaction to the allergen that is causing their symptoms. Remember lymphocytes recirculate within tissues (homing) so an allergen that causes a response when it is ingested may not cause a response on skin testing.

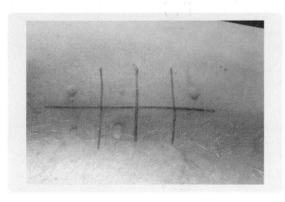

Allergic rhinitis

Nasal congestion, watery nasal discharge and sneezing occur after exposure to allergen. The most common allergens are grass, flower, weed or tree pollens, which cause a seasonal rhinitis (hay fever), and house-dust mite faeces, which can cause a more perennial rhinitis. Allergic attacks usually last for a few hours and are often accompanied by smarting and watering of the eyes. Skin prick tests can identify the allergen.

The most important treatment is topical (nasal) steroids; alternatives or adjuncts include antihistamines or mast cell stabilizers such as sodium cromoglicate. Avoidance of allergens is advised but is often difficult.

Anaphylaxis

Anaphylaxis is a medical emergency and can be fatal. However, it is rapidly reversible if treated properly. A systemic response to an allergen that is either intravenous or rapidly absorbed can cause tracheal occlusion and shock. Many allergens can cause anaphylaxis, but more common causes include drugs, bee stings and peanuts. The signs of anaphylaxis are principally those of shock. Signs include:

- Hypotension with tachycardia
- Warm peripheral temperature
- Signs of airway obstruction
- Laryngeal and facial oedema and urticaria (often seen).

The initial management of anaphylaxis is resuscitation. Allergens should be removed if possible, e.g. stop drug infusion, and the patient should be given high-flow oxygen. Adrenaline (epinephrine) should be given intramuscularly and repeated after 5 minutes if there is no improvement. Adrenaline should be given intravenously only in life-threatening profound shock. Fluids might be needed for patients in shock and a β_2-adrenoreceptor agonist can be used to reverse bronchospasm. People who have had anaphylactic reactions often carry adrenaline with them so that it can be administered rapidly in an emergency. Steroids and antihistamines act too slowly to be effective in anaphylaxis.

AUTOIMMUNITY

Prevention of autoimmunity

Autoimmunity is a state in which the body exhibits immunological reactivity to itself. 'Self-tolerance' is the generic term given to the mechanisms by which T and B cells are prevented from responding to self. Because T and B cells randomly recombine the genes for their receptors, there is a risk of producing receptors that will react with self-antigen. These cells must be eliminated to make the host tolerant to itself.

Central tolerance

Central tolerance is by negative selection—early clonal deletion. T cells (in the thymus) and B cells (in the bone marrow) are eliminated if they are self-reactive. Central tolerance is not complete. Only the most self-reactive lymphocytes are deleted, ensuring that a wide lymphocyte repertoire is maintained.

Peripheral tolerance

In the periphery, self-antigens do not generally elicit an immune response. Several mechanisms prevent self-reactive T cells from causing autoimmune disease, including:

- Lack of the co-stimulatory molecules required for T cell activation, e.g. cells expressing self-antigen do not express CD40 or CD28
- Sequestration of the antigen behind a physical barrier, e.g. the testis
- Lack of antigen presentation, because of low level MHC expression
- T cells entering immune privileged sites undergo apoptosis (via Fas, transforming growth factor (TGF)-β or IL-10). Immune privileged sites include the brain, testis and the anterior chamber of the eye
- A negative feedback system (cytotoxic T lymphocyte antigen 4) prevents overstimulation of an immune response.

Immune regulation
Response to self-antigen can also be regulated by a population of T cells producing suppressive cytokines. Regulatory T cells (T regs) inhibit responses of other T cells through mechanisms that are as yet poorly understood.

Causes of autoimmunity—breakdown of tolerance

If tolerance breaks down, autoimmunity can develop. Tolerance can break down in the thymus (usually for genetic reasons) or in the periphery (usually as a result of environmental factors such as

infection). Autoimmunity is multifactorial; a defect in at least one of the regulatory mechanisms is required before disease develops.

Role of human leucocyte antigen (HLA)—genetic predisposition

Many autoimmune diseases have a familial component. The HLA haplotype is the main identified genetic factor. If an individual has inherited an HLA allele that does not bind self-antigen with high affinity, reactive T cells are not deleted in the thymus. Certain HLA alleles are linked to specific autoimmune processes, e.g. HLA-DR4 in rheumatoid arthritis. However, a certain HLA haplotype does not automatically result in the development of an autoimmune disease; 95% of patients with ankylosing spondylitis have HLA-B27, but only 5% of the population with HLA-B27 have ankylosing spondylitis.

Role of infection—molecular mimicry

Certain bacteria and viruses possess antigens that resemble sequestered host-cell components, and infection with these can generate an immune response against self. An example of molecular mimicry is cross-reactivity between heart muscle and streptococcal antigens, leading to rheumatic fever. This is short-lived and reversible and is not a major cause of autoimmunity.

Role of infection—polyclonal activation

Many infections are able to activate T and B cells in a non-specific fashion. This results in the proliferation of several T and B cell clones, which can produce autoreactive autoantibody or mediate autoimmunity.

Role of infection—inappropriate MHC expression

Infection stimulates antigen-presenting cells, and upregulation of MHC class II molecules can result in activation of autoreactive T cells.

Mechanisms of autoimmunity

Autoimmune diseases are hypersensitivity reactions in which an exaggerated response is triggered by self-antigen. Autoimmune diseases can therefore be classified in the same way as hypersensitivity (excluding type I hypersensitivity).

Antibody-mediated (type II hypersensitivity reactions)

Antibodies that are specific for self-antigen bind to tissues or cells. Autoimmunity can result from a variety of mechanisms, including:

- Opsonization: e.g. in autoimmune haemolytic anaemia, IgG binds to red blood cells, which are phagocytosed by macrophages in the spleen
- Complement activation: e.g. in severe autoimmune haemolytic anaemia, IgM antibodies bound to red blood cells activate complement, resulting in lysis within the circulation.

Neutralization and ADCC can also occur in response to self-antigen.

Immune-complex-mediated (type III hypersensitivity reactions)

Immune complexes are lattices of antigen and antibody. They are usually cleared rapidly from the circulation, but complexes that are not cleared trigger inflammation, particularly in blood vessels. An example of a type III autoimmune disease is SLE. A consequence of the presence of circulating immune complexes can be the development of glomerulonephritis. Immune complexes deposit in the capillaries of the glomerular tufts in the kidneys, resulting in renal failure. Immune complexes are also deposited at other sites, e.g. joints, skin and brain.

Cell-mediated (type IV hypersensitivity reactions)

These comprise autoimmune T cell responses, usually by T helper and T cytotoxic cells. Examples include rheumatoid arthritis and type I diabetes mellitus.

Clinically autoimmunity is divided into systemic (connective tissue diseases and vasculitis) and organ-specific conditions.

Systemic autoimmune diseases

Systemic lupus erythematosus (SLE)

In SLE, the main autoantibodies are directed against DNA, histone proteins, red blood cells, platelets, leucocytes and clotting factors. Diagnosis is by antinuclear antibody testing. It is most commonly diagnosed in women in the second or third decade of life.

The aetiology is unknown but the vast array of autoantibodies present suggests a breakdown of self-tolerance. Genetic factors predispose to the disease. There is an association with HLA-DR2 and HLA-DR3, and with deficiencies of complement proteins, especially C2 or C4 (reduced complement levels result in a decreased ability to clear immune complexes). Other relevant aetiological factors include drugs such as hydralazine, exposure to ultraviolet light and oestrogens.

Deposition of immune complexes leads to the various clinical features of SLE, including:

- Arthritis (deposition in joints)
- Rashes in sun-exposed areas
- Glomerulonephritis.

SLE is treated with immunosuppression, steroids, NSAIDs or other anti-inflammatory drugs.

Rheumatoid arthritis (RA)

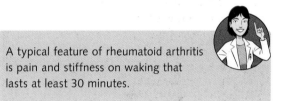

A typical feature of rheumatoid arthritis is pain and stiffness on waking that lasts at least 30 minutes.

RA is a chronic systemic disease that primarily involves the joints, resulting in inflammation of the synovium and destruction of the articular cartilage (Fig. 2.15). Initially, the disease affects the small joints of the hands and feet symmetrically, later spreading to the larger joints. RA affects approximately 1–2% of the world's population and is most common between the ages of 30 and 55 years. The female : male ratio is 3 : 1.

Approximately 70% of RA patients carry either the HLA-DR4 or HLA-DR1 haplotype. The immunopathogenesis of RA is outlined in Fig. 2.16. A key event in RA is secretion of TNF by T cells and macrophages. TNF causes joint inflammation and erosion of bone, and can be blocked by infliximab.

A summary of other systemic connective tissue disorders and vasculitides is given in Figs 2.17 and 2.18.

Fig. 2.15 Rheumatoid joint showing pannus formation and cartilage destruction. The synovial membrane is infiltrated by inflammatory cells and hypertrophies to form granulation tissue known as 'pannus'. This eventually erodes the articular cartilage and bone. T cells and macrophages in the inflamed synovium secrete tumour necrosis factor. PMN, polymorphonuclear neutrophil.

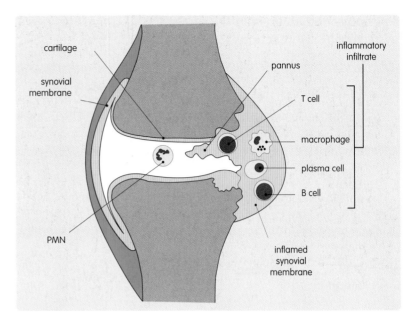

Fig. 2.16 Pathogenesis of rheumatoid arthritis (RA). Autoreactive CD4$^+$ T cells mediate the pathological changes. Synovial T cells produce a number of cytokines including tumour necrosis factor (TNF). These stimulate the acute phase response, synovial inflammation and bone erosion. Activation of B cells can result in the production of rheumatoid factor and immune complex formation.

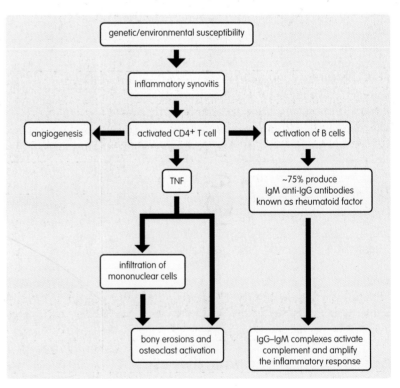

Rheumatoid arthritis

The blood tests in RA reflect its inflammatory nature; CRP and ESR are raised, indicating an acute phase response. Rheumatoid nodules are present when the patient has made IgM anti-IgG autoantibodies (rheumatoid factor) and indicate a poorer prognosis than those who are rheumatoid factor negative.

Radiographic features include:
- Soft tissue swelling
- Juxta-articular osteoporosis
- Joint space narrowing
- Joint destruction and erosions (see photograph)
- Subluxation.

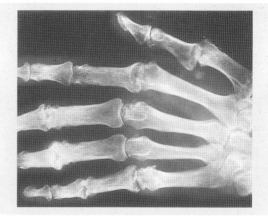

Fig. 2.17 Other autoimmune diseases of connective tissues

Disease	Autoantigen	Diagnostic tests	Features
Sjögren's syndrome	Exocrine glands	Anti-Ro and La	Reduced lacrimal and salivary gland secretion, causing dry eyes and mouth
Myositis	Muscle	ANA (Jo-1)	Muscle weakness and atrophy; mild arthritis and rashes are common
Systemic sclerosis	Nucleoli	ANA (topoisomerase 1 and centromere)	Increased collagen deposition in skin; usually runs an indolent course, but eventual involvement of internal organs occurs in most patients
Mixed connective tissue disease (MCTD)		ANA (RNP)	Features of SLE, RA, scleroderma and polymyositis; may not be a distinct entity

ANA, anti-nuclear antigen; RA, rheumatoid arthritis; RNP, ribonucleoprotein; SLE, systemic lupus erythematosus.

Fig. 2.18 Autoimmune vasculitides

Disease	Diagnostic test	Features
Polyangiitis	p-ANCA (myeloperoxidase)	Necrotizing inflammation of medium-sized arteries. Any organ or tissue can be affected
Wegener's granulomatosis	c-ANCA (proteinase 3)	Presents with respiratory tract lesions, typically in the lungs and nose, in association with glomerulonephritis

Antineutrophil cytoplasmic antibodies (ANCA) are specific antibodies against neutrophils. p-ANCA reacts with neutrophil myeloperoxidase and gives a perinuclear pattern on immunofluorescence; c-ANCA reacts with proteinase 3 in the cytoplasm and gives a diffuse cytoplasmic pattern in immunofluorescence.

Fig. 2.19 Summary of organ-/cell-specific autoimmune (AI) diseases

Disease	Autoantigen	Features
Myasthenia gravis	Acetylcholine receptor	Muscle weakness and fatiguability due to impaired neuromuscular transmission; 70% of patients have thymic hyperplasia, 10% have thymic tumour
Goodpasture's syndrome	Type IV collagen in the basement membrane of kidney and lung	Pulmonary haemorrhage and acute glomerulonephritis; peak incidence in men in their mid-20s
Pernicious anaemia	Intrinsic factor	See p. 86
AI haemolytic anaemia	Erythrocyte membrane antigens	See p. 93
AI thrombocytopenia	Platelet glycoproteins	See p. 114
Hashimoto's thyroiditis	Thyroid peroxidase	See p. 52
Graves' disease	TSH receptor	See p. 52
Type I diabetes mellitus	Islet cell antigens	See below
Coeliac disease	Tissue transglutaminase	Malabsorption due to villous atrophy in the small bowel. Diarrhoea and anaemia are common. Patients can present at any age. Treated with a gluten-free diet

The organ-specific autoantibodies are caused by similar genes, usually in the HLA complex. Family members therefore tend to have different organ-specific diseases. TSH, thyroid stimulating hormone.

Wegener's granulomatosis

Wegener's granulomatosis is a systemic vasculitis (results from blood vessel inflammation) that affects the nose, lungs and kidneys. The pathogenesis of Wegener's is linked to antibodies directed against proteinase-3, an enzyme present in the cytoplasm of neutrophils (c-ANCA). It causes neutrophils to become trapped in vessel walls where they release proinflammatory cytokines and cause damage. The most severe complication is kidney failure; however, the use of immunosuppressives has drastically improved the prognosis.

Organ- or cell-type-specific autoimmune diseases

A summary of organ- or cell-type-specific diseases is given in Fig. 2.19.

Hashimoto's thyroiditis

Hashimoto's thyroiditis is the most common cause of goitrous hypothyroidism. Antigen-specific cytotoxic T cells attack the thyroid gland, leading to progressive destruction of the epithelium. Marked lymphocytic infiltration (mainly by B cells and CD4+ T cells) of the thyroid gland is accompanied by migration of large numbers of macrophages and plasma cells, resulting in the formation of lymphoid follicles and germinal centres within the thyroid. Due to unregulated T-helper cell interaction with B cells, autoantibodies are produced against thyroid antigens such as thyroid peroxidase.

Middle-aged females are most commonly affected (female : male ratio of 5 : 1). The disease is associated with HLA-DR5 and HLA-DR3 haplotypes.

Graves' disease

Graves' disease is the commonest cause of hyperthyroidism. This arises as a result of IgG autoantibody production against the thyroid stimulating hormone receptor that actively stimulates the receptor, resulting in increased thyroxine production.

Graves' disease affects 1–2% of females. The female : male ratio is 5 : 1. There is a strong association with HLA-DR3 in Caucasian people.

Clinical features of Graves' disease

Graves' disease is associated with pretibial oedema and a variety of eye signs (see photograph):
- Exophthalmos
- Lid retraction
- Lid lag
- Ophthalmoplegia
- Conjunctival and periorbital oedema.

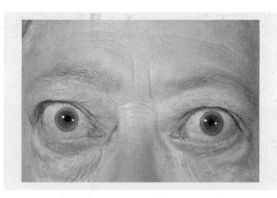

Insulin-dependent (type I) diabetes mellitus

This disorder occurs due to destruction of the insulin-producing β cells of the islets of Langerhans of the pancreas. One in 300 people in Europe and the USA is affected. An autoimmune aetiology is suspected. Over 90% of patients with the disease carry either HLA-DR3 or HLA-DR4 or both. Viral infection is believed to trigger T cells to invade the islets and attack β cells, which are rapidly destroyed.

Antibodies against islet antigens are transiently produced and act as a marker for the process.

IMMUNE DEFICIENCY

Immune deficiency predisposes individuals to infections from opportunistic pathogens (those that do not normally cause disease) as well as normal pathogens. Although the cause of the deficiency can be primary or secondary, the part of the immune system that is deficient will determine the sort of infection to which the individual is predisposed. Antibody deficits result in extracellular bacterial infection. T cell deficiencies can result in viral, fungal and intracellular bacterial infections.

Primary immune deficiencies

Primary immunodeficiencies are intrinsic, usually inherited, defects of the immune system. Different components of the immune system can be affected, including:

- Antibodies (Fig. 2.20)
- T cells (Fig. 2.21)
- Phagocytes (Fig. 2.22)
- Complement (Fig. 2.23).

It is important to recognize primary immunodeficiencies. Patients with an antibody deficiency will develop irreversible lung infections (bronchiectasis) unless given immunoglobulin. Children with T cell defects can be killed by opportunistic infections or from live vaccines such as BCG.

Neonates do not possess a fully developed immune system at birth. In the neonatal period,

Fig. 2.20 Primary antibody deficiencies

Disorder	Features
Transient physiological agammaglobulinaemia of the neonate	See Fig. 2.24
X-linked agammaglobulinaemia of Bruton	X-linked recessive disorder with defective B cell maturation. Low serum immunoglobulin levels result in recurrent pyogenic infections (seen at about 6 months). Treatment is with immunoglobulin replacement
Common variable hypogammaglobulinaemia	Heterogeneous group of disorders with normal lymphocyte numbers but abnormal B cell function; late onset (15–35 years) presenting with recurrent pyogenic infections. Treatment is with immunoglobulin replacement
Selective IgA deficiency	Occurs in 1 in 700 Caucasians but is rare in other ethnic groups; can be asymptomatic or produce recurrent infections of the respiratory and gastrointestinal tracts

Pyogenic infections are common due to infections with encapsulated bacteria such as streptococci and staphylococci (not selective IgA deficiency).

Fig. 2.21 Primary lymphocyte deficiencies

Disorder	Features
DiGeorge syndrome (thymic hypoplasia)	Intrauterine damage to the third and fourth pharyngeal pouches results in failure of development of the thyroid and parathyroid glands. This results in a decrease in the number and function of T cells Clinical features include abnormal facies, cardiac defects, hypoparathyroidism and recurrent infections
Severe combined immunodeficiency disease (SCID)	Lymphocyte deficiency and failure of thymic development due to inherited abnormalities: • X-linked SCID is due to defects in the γ-chain of the IL-2 receptor. The γ-chain forms part part of several cytokine receptors including IL-7, which is needed for T cell maturation • Autosomal recessive SCID is caused by defects in adenosine deaminase (ADA) or purine nucleoside phosphorylase in more than 50% of cases. Both are involved in purine degradation and deficiency results in accumulation of toxic metabolites and inhibition of DNA synthesis. Recombinase defects also lead to SCID In both types of SCID, treatment should be by bone marrow transplant, usually before the age of 2 years. Gene therapy has been used for X-linked SCID, although two cases of leukaemia have occurred
Wiskott–Aldrich syndrome	X-linked recessive condition characterized by normal serum IgG, low IgM and high IgA and IgE. Defective T cell function is seen, which worsens as the patient ages. Patients tend to get recurrent infections, eczema and thrombocytopenia

Primary lymphocyte deficiencies include infections with opportunistic pathogens such as Pneumocystis carinii. *T cell deficiency can cause an antibody deficiency due to lack of T-helper-cell activation of B cells.*

Fig. 2.22 Primary phagocyte deficiencies

Disorder	Features
Neutropenia	See p. 109
Leucocyte adhesion deficiency	Lack of β_2-integrin molecules results in impaired adhesion and extravasation of phagocytes
Chronic granulomatous disease	Most commonly X-linked (can be autosomal recessive) inheritance. Lack of NADPH oxidase (see p. 7) impairs killing of ingested pathogens, which therefore persist. Can be tested by impaired reduction of nitroblue tetrazolium by stimulated neutrophils

NADPH, nicotinamide adenine dinucleotide phosphate.

Fig. 2.23 Primary complement deficiencies

Disorder	Features
Deficiency of classical pathway components	Tend to develop immune complex disease
C3 deficiency	Prone to recurrent pyogenic infections
Deficiency of C5, C6, C7, C8, factor D, properdin	Increased susceptibility to *Neisseria* infections
C1 inhibitor deficiency	Causes hereditary angioedema

Deficiencies of almost all complement components have been described.

infants are normally protected by maternal IgG that crossed the placenta in utero, but this is metabolized during the first months of life. Infants normally begin production of their own IgG by 3 months (Fig. 2.24). In some individuals, IgG production might not start for up to 9–12 months, possibly due to lack of help from T cells.

Secondary immune deficiencies

Malnutrition and disease

Rarely, lack of dietary protein and certain elements (e.g. zinc) predisposes to secondary immunodeficiency. Infections such as malaria and measles also result in immunodeficiency.

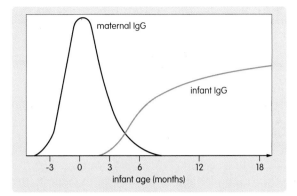

Fig. 2.24 Plasma levels of maternal and neonatal immunoglobulin in the normal-term infant. In the first 6 months of life there is a trough in immunoglobulin levels that makes infants prone to infection. IgA in breast milk can compensate. Babies born prematurely are deprived of maternal IgG and suffer exaggerated neonatal antibody deficiency.

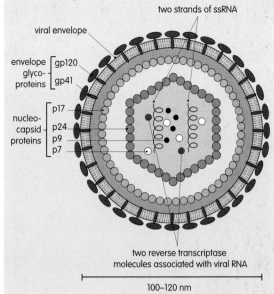

Fig. 2.25 Structure of HIV-1. The envelope glycoproteins gp120 and gp41 are hypervariable. gp120 binds CD4, allowing entry of the virus into the cell. The viral envelope is a lipid bilayer containing both viral glycoprotein antigens and host proteins.

Malignancy

Secondary immunodeficiency is particularly common with tumours that arise from the immune system, such as myeloma, lymphoma and leukaemia (see Chapter 5). Many other tumours are immunosuppressive. This is likely to provide the tumour cells with a selective advantage, because they evade destruction by cytotoxic cells.

Steroids, other drugs and radiation

Iatrogenic causes of immunosuppression are common. Immunosuppressive drugs can be given to suppress inflammatory or autoimmune disease, or to prevent rejection of transplanted material (see p. 60). Radiation and cytotoxic drugs can be used to treat malignancies and frequently cause immunosuppression.

Acquired immunodeficiency syndrome (AIDS)

AIDS is caused by infection with HIV. HIV is a retrovirus, containing a small amount of RNA that codes three important viral genes: the envelope, reverse transcriptase and protease (Fig. 2.25).

The envelope is composed of gp120 which binds to CD4 receptors and chemokine receptor 5 (CC5), allowing HIV to infect:

- CD4 T cells
- Monocytes and macrophages
- Dendritic cells.

Reverse transcriptase is an enzyme that catalyses the production of HIV DNA from RNA using host cellular machinery.

Protease is an enzyme that cleaves proteins into their component peptides, and is important for viral assembly and activity.

Transmission of HIV

Sexual transmission is the most important route for spread; HIV infects mucosal macrophages and dendritic cells via CD4 and CC5. These professional APCs then aid in the evolution of the HIV infection by transporting them to the lymph nodes where HIV can gain easy access to CD4 T helper cells.

Transmission can also occur through infected blood: blood transfusions, intravenous drug abusers and needlestick injury (0.3% risk from a single exposure). These routes do not require HIV to gain access through mucous membranes and hence CC5 receptors. Vertical transmission is especially important in developing countries, occurring transplacentally during labour (approximately 25% of cases) or through breast milk.

Immune response to HIV

Most individuals exposed to HIV sexually become chronically infected. Sterilizing immunity is very rare. Infected individuals produce antibody, but this is largely ineffective against intracellular virus. T cells inhibit HIV (by interferon secretion) or kill infected cells.

The primary infection is often asymptomatic but may be marked by a flu-like illness (fever, macular rash, mouth ulcers, splenomegaly and diarrhoea) in 15% of individuals.

> **HIV seroconversion illness**
>
> Individuals infected with HIV develop symptoms as their body starts to produce antibody to HIV. This is called HIV seroconversion illness. The patient experiences fever, rash, malaise, sore throat, diarrhoea and arthralgia; lymphadenopathy may also be present. Not all patients experience seroconversion illness, and it is often diagnosed retrospectively.

How does HIV progress to AIDS?

1. Mutations: reverse transcriptase makes an error for roughly 1 in every 10,000 bases. Some of these mutations provide a selective advantage to the HIV, e.g. cells of the immune system may no longer recognize them, and another immune response has to start afresh.
2. Even if the immune system manages to clear the entire free virus, HIV can hide in host DNA and remain dormant for many years— the latent phase. Reactivation of the host cell then results in production of HIV RNA, and thus the infection continues.
3. HIV infects and destroys the cells that are responsible for the immune response. As the CD4 count declines, the cytotoxic T lymphocytes become less effective as they are receiving less support from T helper cells.

> Each infected individual contains many hundreds of slightly different strains following infection with a single virus.

Diagnosis and monitoring of an HIV infection

Screening for HIV infection is performed using ELISAs to detect anti-HIV antibodies. If the ELISA is positive, confirmatory tests must be carried out, e.g. a Western blot, which detects antibodies against specific HIV proteins. As seroconversion (production of antibodies) might not take place until 3 months after infection, there is a window period when ELISA will be negative. This is a potential problem in blood transfusion (see p. 127).

In infants, anti-HIV IgG can be maternally derived and persist for up to 18 months, making diagnosis of HIV by ELISA unreliable. Detection of HIV by polymerase chain reaction (PCR) is used to confirm HIV infection in neonates.

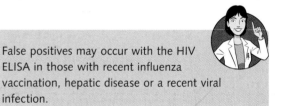

> False positives may occur with the HIV ELISA in those with recent influenza vaccination, hepatic disease or a recent viral infection.

Determinations of CD4 T cell counts and measurement of the viral load (serum HIV RNA) are useful in assessing response to treatment and the prognosis.

CD4 counts provide a guide of the current immunological status of the patient (Fig. 2.26), whereas HIV RNA levels predict what will happen to the patient over the next few months and years.

During the latent phase of the infection T cells are constantly battling with the HIV, and gradually the CD4 count falls. With the falling CD4 count, individuals become susceptible to more and more organisms. Initially these include virulent organisms such as *Candida albicans* and *Mycobacterium tuberculosis*. When the CD4 count drops to <200 cells/µL, the individual becomes susceptible to opportunistic infections such as *Pneumocystis carinii* pneumonia, a reflection of severe immunodeficiency (Fig. 2.27).

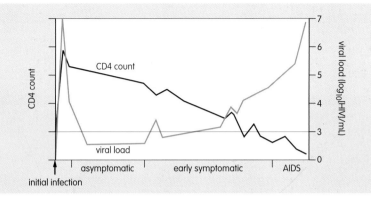

Fig. 2.26 Variation in CD4 count and viral load during the course of HIV infection.

Fig. 2.27 Clinical infections at different CD4 counts

CD4 count	Infection
<400	Tuberculosis
<300	Kaposi's sarcoma Oesophageal candidiasis
<200	*Pneumocystis carinii* pneumonia (PCP) Toxoplasmosis
<100	*Mycobacterium avium intracellulare* Cytomegalovirus retinitis

Individuals should have their CD4 and viral load levels checked every 3–6 months.

Treatment of HIV

The treatment of HIV is now very successful. Although the infection cannot be cured, survival and quality of life have been profoundly increased. The drugs used to combat the virus are termed antiretrovirals and include classes of drug that work on the three main elements of the virus—the envelope, reverse transcriptase and protease (see p. 55) (Fig. 2.28).

When treating HIV it is important to remember its ability to mutate and that antiretrovirals could provide a selective advantage for a more resistant strain to develop. For this reason a combination of a least two classes of drug are used and they are not started until there is evidence of CD4 T cell decline.

Antibiotic prophylaxis against infections such as *Pneumocystis carinii* and *Toxoplasma gondii* is effective and usually given when the CD4 count is <200/μL. It has been shown that antibiotic prophylaxis can be safely stopped following immune restoration using treatment with antiretroviral therapy.

IMMUNIZATION

Concepts of immunization

It is important to be able to explain the difference between active and passive immunity. Active immunity is produced by the body in response to antigen (either infection or vaccination). In vaccination, active immunity produces a response to antigen that is given to the patient. Preformed antibodies are used in passive immunization.

Immunity can be achieved by passive or active immunization (Fig. 2.29).

Passive immunization

This is a temporary immunity that results from the transfer of exogenous antibody and thus occurs without prior exposure to the specific antigens. Passive immunity is seen in the fetus when maternal IgG crosses the placenta and in breast-fed babies due to the IgA content of breast milk. Passive immunity can be conferred to individuals exposed to a

Fig. 2.28 Antiretroviral agents in current use and their site of action in the lifecycle of HIV. AZT, azidothymidine.

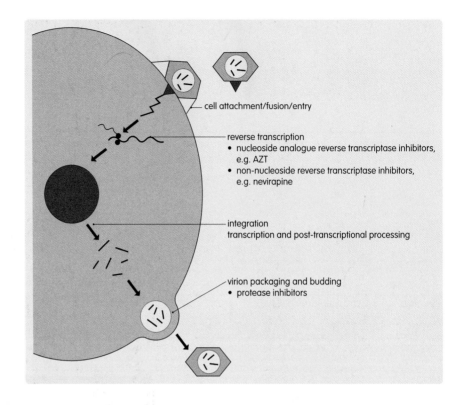

- cell attachment/fusion/entry

- reverse transcription
  - nucleoside analogue reverse transcriptase inhibitors, e.g. AZT
  - non-nucleoside reverse transcriptase inhibitors, e.g. nevirapine

- integration
  transcription and post-transcriptional processing

- virion packaging and budding
  - protease inhibitors

Fig. 2.29 Comparison of passive and active immunity

	Passive	Active
Features	Preformed immunoglobulins transferred to individual	Contact with antigen induces adaptive immune response
	Large amounts of antibody available immediately	Takes some time to develop immunity
	Short lifespan of antibodies	Long-lived immunity induced
Examples	Antitetanus toxin antibody	Natural exposure; vaccination

pathogen to which they are not immune by the injection of immunoglobulins to the antigen, taken from blood donors immune to the pathogen, e.g. a non-immunized patient exposed to hepatitis B would benefit from this kind of postinfection prophylaxis.

Examples where passive immunity is used:
- Prevent hepatitis A and B infection
- Prevent varicella zoster
- Treat snake bites (anti-venom).

Active immunization

Active immunization results from contact with antigens, either through natural infection or by vaccination. Individuals exhibit a primary immune response, with clonal expansion of B and T cells and formation of memory cells. Subsequent exposure to the same antigen will induce a secondary immune response (see p. 20).

Vaccination

Vaccination is a form of active immunization that induces specific immunity to a particular pathogen. The aim is to produce a rapid, protective immune response on re-exposure to that pathogen. An ideal vaccine is:

- Safe, with minimal side-effects and free from contaminating substances
- Immunogenic, activating the required branches of the immune system, inducing long-lasting local and systemic immunity
- Heat stable, because there are difficulties with refrigeration, particularly in tropical countries

- Inexpensive, an important consideration, especially in developing countries.

Types of vaccine

The types of vaccine in current use are listed in Fig. 2.30. Vaccines are live attenuated, killed or subunit; the features of each are compared in Fig. 2.31. The routine immunization schedule used in the UK is shown in Fig. 2.32.

Fig. 2.30 Different types of vaccine in use in the UK today

Vaccine	Features	Examples
Live attenuated	Attenuation achieved by repeated culture on artificial media or by serial passage in animals; immunogenicity is retained, but virulence is significantly diminished	Oral polio (Sabin), BCG, rubella, measles, mumps (MMR)
Killed	Intact organisms killed by exposure to heat or chemicals, e.g. formalin	Intramuscular polio (Salk), pertussis, influenza
Subunit	Purified, protective immunity-inducing antigenic components; often surface antigens	Non-conjugated pneumococcal, non-conjugated *Haemophilus*
Recombinant	Genes encoding epitopes, which elicit protective immunity, are inserted into pro- or eukaryotic cells; large quantities of vaccine are produced rapidly	Hepatitis B surface antigen (produced in yeast cells)
Toxoids	Bacterial toxins inactivated by heat or chemicals	Diphtheria, tetanus
Conjugates	Polysaccharide antigen is linked to protein carrier to enhance Immunogenicity	*Haemophilus influenzae* type B (Hib), meningococcal, pneumococcal

BCG, bacille Calmette–Guérin.

Fig. 2.31 Features of live versus killed vaccines

Feature	Live attenuated vaccine	Killed vaccine
Level of immunity induced	High: organism replicates at site of infection (mimicking natural infection)	Low: non-replicating organisms produce a short-lived stimulus
Cell-mediated response	Good: antigens are processed and presented with MHC molecules	Poor
Local immunity	Good	Poor
Cost	Expensive to produce and administer	Cheaper than live vaccines
Reversion to virulence	Possible but rare	No (therefore safe for immunocompromised and pregnant patients)
Stability	Heat labile	Heat stable
Risk of contamination	Possible, e.g. by virus in cell media	N/A

The genes of attenuated organisms can differ from the wild type by just a few base pairs. It is relatively easy for them to mutate back to the disease-causing str ain. MHC, major histocompatibility complex; N/A, not applicable.

Fig. 2.32 Routine immunization schedule used in the UK

Age	Vaccine
Neonate (certain groups)	BCG
2, 3, 4 months	Diphtheria/tetanus/pertussis (DTP) Polio Hib Meningococcus C
12–15 months	MMR
4–5 years	MMR, diphtheria, tetanus, acellular pertussis
13–18 years	Boosters for diphtheria, tetanus, oral polio
Adult	Boosters for tetanus and polio Occupational or lifestyle risk
65 years	Influenza
Any age	Influenza, pneumococcus Occupation Hep A, Hep B Travel, e.g. Yellow fever

This schedule is set to change with pneumococcal vaccination to be added to the injections received by infants.

It is possible to enhance the immune response to vaccines by using adjuvants. Adjuvants, e.g. aluminium salts and *Bordetella pertussis*, are non-specific.

Vaccines are not 100% efficacious. A small proportion of individuals receiving vaccination will not respond adequately. However, by immunizing the majority of the population, non-responders are unlikely to come into contact with the virus because the viral reservoir is reduced (herd immunity).

Vaccination against toxins such as tetanus does not provide immunity against the toxin-producing bacterium (*Clostridium tetani*). Its benefits come from preventing the sequelae associated with the tetanus toxin, i.e. tetanus of the masseter muscles (lock jaw).

You will notice that a number of vaccinations are given simultaneously; this is not just for convenience. Given alone some of the subunit vaccines would not evoke a sufficient immune response in order for immunity to develop. For example, the DTP vaccination relies strongly on the danger signal produced in response to the killed pertussis organism to develop immunity to the diphtheria and tetanus toxoids.

TRANSPLANTATION

Mechanisms of solid organ transplant rejection

Autologous grafts are grafts moved from one part of the body to another, e.g. skin grafts.
Syngeneic grafts are between genetically identical individuals, e.g. monozygotic twins.
Allogeneic grafts are between individuals of the same species.
Xenogeneic grafts are between different species.

Unless the donor and recipient are immunologically identical, the recipient will mount a rejection response against 'foreign' antigens expressed by the graft. The most important graft antigens responsible for an immune response in the recipient are the MHC molecules (see p. 15). However, even when the donor and recipient are genetically identical at the MHC loci, graft rejection can occur due to differences at other loci, which encode minor histocompatibility antigens. A rejection response can lead to loss of a graft. There are three types of graft rejection (Fig. 2.33):

1. Hyperacute: occurs within hours as a result of preformed antibodies, type II hypersensitivity reaction
2. Acute cellular: takes several days to develop, type IV hypersensitivity reaction
3. Chronic: occurs months to years after transplantation; can be caused by a variety of mechanisms.

Fig. 2.33 Patterns of graft rejection

Type	Mechanism	Prevention
Hyperacute (minutes–hours)	Pre-existing antidonor antibodies	Perform cross-match of donor cells and recipient's serum, check for ABO compatibility
Acute cellular (days–weeks)	T cell mediated	HLA matching of donor and recipient, antirejection therapy
Chronic (months–years)	Unclear	HLA matching

HLA, human leucocyte antigen.

Fig. 2.34 Common transplants

Transplant	Notes
Kidney	Live or cadaveric donor; the fewer the MHC mismatches, the greater the success rate; must be ABO compatible
Heart	Matching is beneficial, but often time is a more pressing concern
Liver	No evidence to suggest that matching affects graft survival; rejection less aggressive than for other organs
Skin graft	Most grafts are autologous, but allografts can be used to protect burns patients
Corneal graft	Matching (class II MHC) is required only if a previous graft was vascularized
Stem cell	Host-versus-graft (HVG) or graft-versus-host (GVH) responses possible. The transplant must be well matched and antirejection therapy used. Host immune cells are destroyed by irradiation prior to transplant (avoids HVG). T cells are depleted from the graft (avoids GVH) using monoclonal antibody and complement

Strategies for preventing rejection

HLA typing and antibody cross-matching

The ideal match is that between monozygotic twins. In all other situations there will be some genetic disparity between donor and recipient. The aim of matching is to minimize genetic differences between donor and recipient. Both the donor and recipient will be HLA typed.

Antirejection therapy

Immunosuppressive drugs can be used to prevent rejection by suppressing antibody and T cell responses. Examples of drugs used include:

- Steroids: these are anti-inflammatory (see p. 42)
- Azathioprine and mycophenolate mofetil: antiproliferative drugs
- Tacrolimus, ciclosporin and rapamycin: inhibit signalling in T cells.

The disadvantage of such non-specific therapy is that the recipient is at increased risk of opportunistic infections (e.g. cytomegalovirus) and certain malignancies. Newer, more selective agents are being developed, including anti-CD3 and anti-IL-2 receptor monoclonal antibodies.

Common types of transplantation performed today are summarized in Fig. 2.34.

Stem cell transplant

Stem cell transplants are used in the treatment of some cancers and primary immunodeficiencies. Stem cells are obtained from bone marrow or blood. Imperfectly matched stem cells can be rejected by the recipient. In addition, stem cells give rise to lymphocytes, which can attack the host, causing acute or chronic graft-versus-host disease.

HAEMATOLOGY

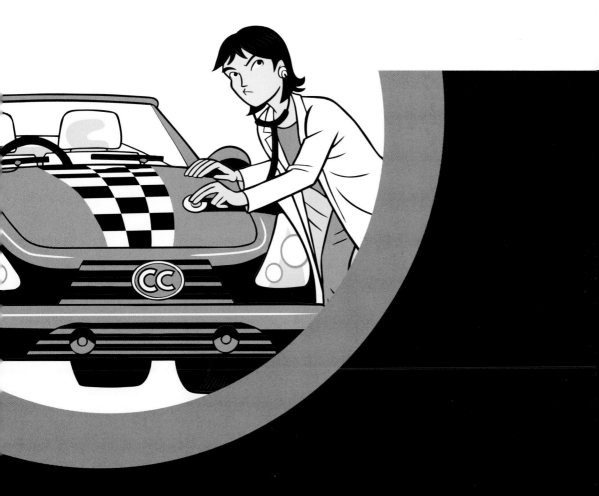

Principles of haematology

Objectives

You should be able to:

- Understand the different components that make up blood
- Describe where and how blood cells are generated
- Know the regulatory factors involved in haemopoiesis
- Know the structure and function of bone marrow and the spleen
- Discuss disorders involving the spleen

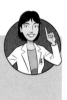

Haematology is a branch of medicine dealing with blood, blood-forming organs and diseases of the blood.

The second part of this book covers haematology, and is organized around the various cell types. The production of blood cells, bone marrow and the function of the spleen are discussed in this chapter. Chapter 4 looks more closely at oxygen transport and the clinical importance of red blood cells. This is followed by the function and clinical relevance of white blood cells. The last three chapters explore haemostasis, including platelets, important blood transfusion and haematological investigations.

OVERVIEW OF HAEMATOLOGY—THE CELL LINES

All blood cells are derived from a pluripotent stem cell, through a process known as haemopoiesis. These stem cells have two important properties: self-renewal and proliferation, and differentiation into progenitor cells committed to a specific cell line. Each of the cells produced has important roles; these are summarized as follows:

Red blood cells
- **Erythrocytes:** utilize haemoglobin to transport oxygen and carbon dioxide between the lungs and the rest of the body (see Chapter 4).

White blood cells (for immune functions see Chapter 1; for cytological appearance, see Chapter 5)

- **Neutrophils:** phagocytose foreign material or dead/damaged cells at sites of inflammation and activate bactericidal mechanisms, produce mediators of chemotaxis
- **Eosinophils:** have all the functions of a neutrophil and are important in the host defence against parasites (coated in antibody). They also regulate immediate hypersensitivity reactions
- **Basophils:** represent the source of most histamine in the human body and can become coated in IgE and release histamine; they mediate type I hypersensitivity reactions. Mast cells in tissues are very similar to basophils in blood
- **Monocytes:** enter tissues to become macrophages. Monocyte-derived cells are found throughout the body as part of the reticuloendothelial system. They phagocytose pathogens and cellular debris and produce various cytokines. They also process and present antigen to lymphocytes as part of the adaptive immune response. Highly specialized mononuclear cells called dendritic cells excel in presenting antigen to T cells
- **B lymphocytes:** as plasma cells they are responsible for immunoglobulin production. They can also become memory B cells
- **T lymphocytes:** cytotoxic CD8 T cells kill cells infected by intracellular organisms. CD4 T helper cells produce cytokines to activate B cells or macrophages

- **Natural killer (NK) cells:** kill cells they detect as foreign either directly or via antibody-dependent cell-mediated cytotoxicity
- **Platelets:** megakaryocyte fragments involved in the haemostatic response to vascular injury by adhering to subendothelial connective tissue (see Chapter 6).

HAEMOPOIESIS AND ITS REGULATION

Haemopoiesis is the formation and development of blood cells. The haemopoietic system is composed of the bone marrow, spleen, liver, lymph nodes and thymus. This process depends upon stem cells, which divide to leave both a reserve population and cells committed to differentiating into the various blood cell lines (Fig. 3.1). Differentiation occurs along one of two lineages:

1. Lymphoid → B and T lymphocytes and NK cells
2. Non-lymphoid → erythrocytes, neutrophils, basophils, eosinophils, monocytes and megakaryocytes.

Sites of haemopoiesis

The main site of haemopoiesis changes during fetal development and maturation:

- Conception to 6 weeks: fetal yolk sac
- 6 weeks to 6 months: fetal liver and spleen
- 6 months onwards: bone marrow.

Progenitor cells

In vitro, haemopoietic progenitors are detected via assays that identify cells capable of producing colonies (a colony-forming unit, or CFU). Granulocytes, erythrocytes, monocytes and megakaryocytes are

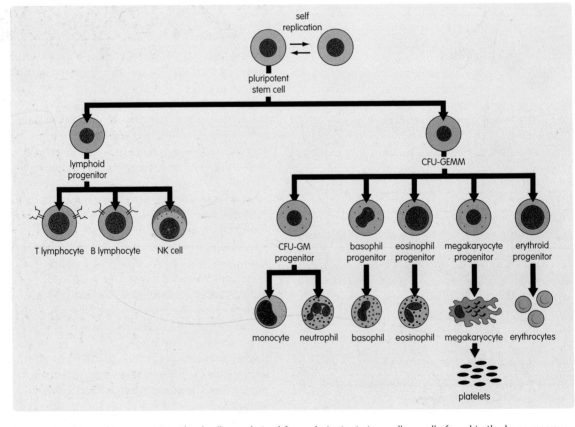

Fig. 3.1 Overview of haemopoiesis. Blood cells are derived from pluripotent stem cells usually found in the bone marrow. Exposure to different growth factors promotes the development of the different cell lines. CFU-GEMM, granulocyte, erythrocyte, monocyte, megakaryocyte colony-forming unit; CFU-GM, granulocyte, monocyte colony-forming unit; NK, natural killer.

produced from a precursor known as CFU-GEMM (also called multipotent myeloid stem cell). This divides into an erythroid progenitor (BFU-E), a megakaryocyte precursor, an eosinophil precursor and a granulocyte/monocyte precursor (CFU-GM). Lymphoid precursors become B cells or NK cells in the bone marrow or travel to the thymus where they develop into T cells.

Regulation of haemopoiesis

Growth factors regulate the balance between haemopoiesis and apoptosis (ageing cells die continually). They also react to external stresses, including infection or blood loss, to maintain or increase the necessary cell types (Fig. 3.2). Growth factors are glycoproteins produced in the bone marrow, liver and kidneys. Binding of the growth factor to surface receptors can trigger replication, differentiation or functional activation; in the absence of stimulation by growth factors, cells undergo apoptosis. Following stimulation by interleukin-1 (IL-1) or tumour necrosis factor (TNF), stromal cells in the bone marrow produce many growth factors. Several growth factors, known as colony-stimulating factors (CSFs), have been identified:

- Multilineage CSF (IL-3): acts early in haemopoiesis to induce non-lymphoid cell production
- Granulocyte–macrophage CSF: acts later on the same cells
- Macrophage CSF and granulocyte CSF: are involved later still to produce monocytes and neutrophils.

> **Growth factors**
>
> Growths factors produced using recombinant DNA techniques can be used clinically. For example, erythropoietin (EPO) can be given to treat anaemia in kidney failure. Patients who have undertaken chemotherapy regimens can benefit from administration of CSFs, including G-CSF and GM-CSF, aiding the bone marrow to recover following chemotherapy.

BONE MARROW

Bone marrow is the major haemopoietic organ in the adult human, and is divided into red and yellow bone marrow. The red marrow is where haemopoiesis takes place and is restricted to the central skeleton (sternum, vertebrae, ribs, hip bones, clavicles and lower skull) and the proximal ends of long bones. Although the yellow marrow is essentially a fat store, acting as an energy reserve, in situations where the rate of haemopoiesis needs to increase dramatically, yellow marrow can convert back to red. In a similar manner, should the need arise, the liver and spleen can also resume their fetal haemopoietic role (this can be seen in chronic anaemias).

Structure

The red marrow provides a suitable microenvironment for stem cell growth and development. It has two main components:

1. Specialized fibroblasts, known as adventitial reticular cells, which secrete a framework of reticulin fibres (fine collagen fibres), forming a meshwork that is essential to support developing blood cells
2. A network of blood sinusoids, lined by a single layer of endothelial cells, which interconnect

Fig. 3.2 Growth factors in haemopoiesis

Factor	Site of action
Stem cell factor	Pluripotent cells
IL-3	CFU-GEMM
GM-CSF	CFU-GM
G-CSF	Granulocyte precursor
M-CSF	Monocyte precursor
IL-5	Eosinophil progenitors
Erythropoietin	Erythrocyte progenitors
Thrombopoietin	Megakaryocyte progenitors
IL-6	B cell precursors
IL-2	T cell precursors
IL-1 and TNF	Stromal cells

CFU-GEMM, granulocyte, erythrocyte, monocyte, megakaryocyte colony-forming unit; CFU-GM, granulocyte, monocyte colony-forming unit; G-CSF, granulocyte colony-stimulating factor; GM-CSF, granulocyte–macrophage colony-stimulating factor; IL, interleukin; M-CSF, macrophage colony-stimulating factor; TNF, tumour necrosis factor.

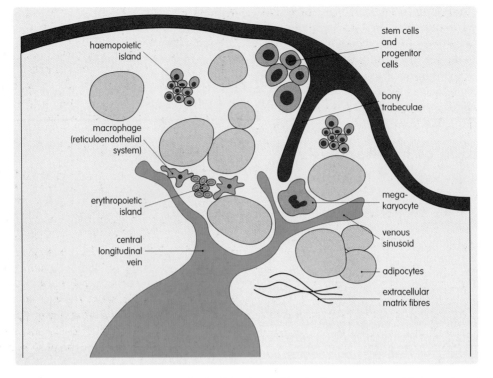

Fig. 3.3 Bone marrow structure. Haemopoietic islands of developing blood cells are interspersed between bony trabeculae and fat cells. A connective tissue stroma of reticular cells and fibres supports the developing cells. Venous plexuses, draining into a central longitudinal vein, transport developed cells out of the bone marrow.

via tight junctions. The vascular sinuses support the haemopoietic cells. They drain into a large central sinus that channels the blood into the systemic venous circulation. The endothelium of the sinusoids exhibits transient cytoplasmic pores, which allow passage of newly formed cells into the circulation.

Haemopoiesis takes place in haemopoietic cords or islands located between the vascular sinuses (Fig. 3.3). Macrophages found within the haemopoietic cords at the centre of each focal group contain stored iron in the form of ferritin and haemosiderin. They have three main functions:

1. Transfer of iron to developing erythroblasts for haemoglobin synthesis
2. Phagocytosis of the cellular debris of haemopoiesis
3. Regulation of haemopoietic cell differentiation and maturation.

Generation of B cells

Bone marrow is considered to be a primary lymphoid organ, i.e. it generates lymphocytes. B-cell development is dependent on stromal cells in the bone marrow. The stroma forms specific adhesion contacts with pro-B cells. As B cells develop, they migrate towards the central axis of the marrow cavity and become less dependent on stromal contact. Immature B cells that bind to self cell-surface antigen are removed from the repertoire at this stage. B cells move to the spleen or lymph nodes for final maturation. T lymphocyte precursors leave the bone marrow early in development and are transferred to the thymus for maturation.

THE SPLEEN

The spleen is a secondary lymphoid organ. It is the site of B and T cell proliferation and of antibody formation, and an important component of the reticuloendothelial system. It is specialized to filter blood, much as the lymph nodes filter lymph, and is a major site of immune response to blood-borne antigens. Blood supply to the spleen is via the splenic artery. Blood is drained via the splenic veins, which join the superior mesenteric vein to form the portal vein.

The spleen is an intraperitoneal organ; its relations comprise:

- Anteriorly: the stomach, tail of the pancreas and left colic flexure
- Medially: the left kidney
- Posteriorly: the diaphragm, and ribs 9–11.

Structure

The spleen is surrounded by a dense, irregular, fibroelastic connective tissue capsule that projects fibres, known as trabeculae, into the organ. The two main types of tissue found within the spleen are red pulp and white pulp. These are separated by a marginal zone (Fig. 3.4).

Red pulp

The red pulp is made up of venous sinuses and splenic cords. The splenic cords are composed of reticular fibres. This region predominantly contains erythrocytes but has a large number of macrophages and dendritic cells. The red pulp removes old or defective erythrocytes and platelets from the circulation.

White pulp and marginal zone

The central arteriole is surrounded by a periarteriolar lymphoid sheath (PALS) which predominantly contains T cells. These branch between B cell follicles that could be primary (unstimulated) but will be secondary (stimulated) in most patients. The PALS and follicles constitute the white pulp. The white pulp is surrounded by a marginal zone containing plasma cells, T and B lymphocytes, macrophages and dendritic cells. The marginal zone is supplied by venous sinuses that have gaps as wide as 2–3 μm between the endothelial cells. The following functions occur in the marginal zone:

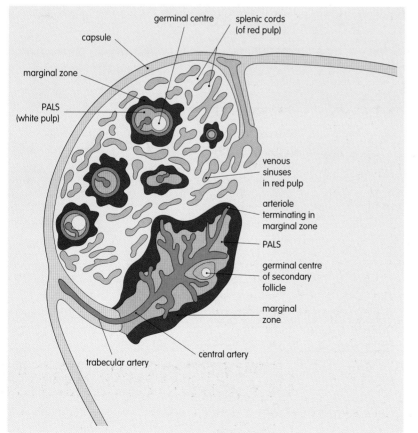

Fig. 3.4 Structure of the spleen. Arterioles entering the spleen are surrounded by T lymphocytes, the periarteriolar lymphoid sheath (PALS). Along with B cells organized into follicles, this constitutes the white pulp. These structures are surrounded by a marginal zone containing plasma cells, lymphocytes, macrophages and dendritic cells. The rest of the spleen is composed of splenic cords (red pulp) and venous sinuses.

- Antigen-presenting cells sample blood for antigens
- Lymphocytes exit the circulation and migrate to their respective domains
- Monocytes enter the spleen and become macrophages. Here they can attack blood-borne microorganisms
- Lymphocytes and dendritic cells come into contact, allowing initiation of an immune response.

The spleen also acts as a reservoir for platelets, erythrocytes and granulocytes.

Embryology

The spleen begins as a mesodermal proliferation in the primitive gut during the fifth week of fetal development. It is connected to the body wall by the lienorenal ligament and to the stomach by the gastrolienal ligament.

Disorders of the spleen
Splenomegaly

Enlargement of the spleen—splenomegaly—is a frequent clinical finding that can occur in a number of different disorders (Fig. 3.5). The causes of splenomegaly are subject to geographical variation; haemolytic disorders predominate in the UK whereas parasitic causes are very common in tropical countries.

The spleen must increase significantly in size in order for it to be palpated below the costal margins; thus a palpable splenic edge always indicates splenomegaly.

Fig. 3.5 Causes of splenomegaly

Category	Type	Causes
Haematological		Lymphomas and leukaemias Polycythaemia rubra vera Haemolytic anaemias Haemoglobinopathies
Infectious	Acute	Infectious mononucleosis Typhoid fever Toxoplasmosis Bacterial endocarditis
	Chronic	Tuberculosis Brucellosis Syphilis Chronic bacteraemia Histoplasmosis
	Parasitic	Malaria Schistosomiasis Leishmaniasis Echinococcosis Trypanosomiasis
Portal hypertension		Liver cirrhosis Cardiac failure (right sided) Hepatic, portal or splenic vein thrombosis
Immunological		Rheumatoid arthritis Felty's syndrome (hypersplenism in rheumatoid arthritis) Systemic lupus erythematosus Sarcoidosis
Storage diseases		Gaucher's disease Niemann–Pick disease
Others		Malignancies (rare) Cysts Amyloid Hyperthyroidism

Congestive splenomegaly

Congestive splenomegaly is caused by persistent venous congestion. Systemic, prehepatic and hepatic causes are the most important.

Splenic infarction

Splenic infarction is relatively common and is caused by the occlusion of the splenic artery or its major branches. Emboli are the most common cause but local thrombi caused by sickle-cell disease and myeloproliferative disorders also occur. Infarcts might be single or multiple. Splenic atrophy can also occur in association with coeliac disease and dermatitis herpetiformis. If the infarction is complete (sometimes referred to as autosplenectomy), patients are rendered functionally asplenic and require the same precautions as other asplenic patients discussed below.

Congenital abnormalities

Congenital asplenia (absence of the spleen) is relatively rare and usually occurs in conjunction with other congenital abnormalities. Approximately 10% of the population have accessory spleens, i.e. additional small areas of splenic tissue.

Rupture of the spleen

Causes include:

- Haemopoietic disorders, e.g. myelofibrosis
- Abdominal trauma, e.g. road traffic accidents
- Infections, e.g. infectious mononucleosis (rare).

Splenectomy

Indications for splenectomy (removal of the spleen) include:

- Severe splenic trauma
- Splenic cysts
- Treatment of idiopathic thrombocytopenic purpura
- Treatment of autoimmune or other types of haemolysis
- Tumours of the spleen and adjacent organs.

Following splenectomy, the patient should be encouraged to mobilize as soon as possible because they are at high risk of thrombosis. There is a life-long increased risk of infection for all individuals without a functioning spleen, particularly with encapsulated organisms (e.g. *Neisseria meningitides, Streptococcus pneumoniae, Haemophilus influenzae*). Management should thus include the following:

- Pneumococcal vaccine should be given (preferably more than 2 weeks before surgery), with boosters every 5–10 years
- Hib and meningococcal vaccine should also be given
- Lifelong prophylactic antibiotics are recommended
- Standby antibiotic should be kept by the patient, to start if any symptoms of infection develop
- Patients should be warned that tropical infections (e.g. malaria) are more likely to be severe
- Urgent hospital admission if infection develops.

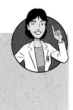

All asplenic patients should be treated in a similar manner, regardless of the cause of their asplenia (splenectomy, autosplenectomy, congenital).

Red blood cells and haemoglobin

Objectives

You should be able to:

- Know the structure and function of red blood cells
- Outline the process of erythropoiesis, including the functions of erythropoietin
- Discuss iron uptake, transport and excretion
- Know the structure and function of haemoglobin and be able to interpret dissociation curves
- Know the different metabolic pathways active in red blood cells
- Have a good understanding of the different types of anaemia
- Distinguish iron deficiency from anaemia of chronic disease
- Understand the physiology of haemoloysis
- Understand the aetiology of sickle cell anaemia and thalassaemia
- Know the different forms of polycythaemia.

STRUCTURE AND FUNCTION OF ERYTHROCYTES

Erythrocyte structure

Erythrocytes are mature red cells with an average lifespan of 120 days (Fig. 4.1). The normal concentration of erythrocytes in the blood is $3.9–6.5 \times 10^{12}$/L. Erythrocytes:

- Are not nucleated and contain no organelles
- Contain millions of molecules of haemoglobin, an oxygen-carrying pigment that gives blood its red colour
- Have a characteristic biconcave discoid shape on blood smears. This gives a 20–30% larger surface area than a sphere of the same volume
- Have an average diameter of 7.2 μm
- Are highly flexible and deform readily, allowing passage through vessels of the microvasculature only 3 μm in diameter.

Erythrocyte function

The primary function of erythrocytes is carriage of oxygen (O_2) and carbon dioxide (CO_2) between the lungs and tissues. The large surface area facilitates this function. They also play an important role in pH buffering.

Gas exchange and transport

The body's resting requirement for O_2 is 250 mL/min. About 200 mL of oxygen is transported in each litre of blood. Multiplied by resting cardiac output (~5 L/min), this means that 1000 mL of O_2 is transported each minute. A small amount of O_2 is dissolved in the blood but the majority is transported by haemoglobin. The oxygen content of the blood depends on three factors:

1. The concentration of haemoglobin
2. The affinity of haemoglobin for oxygen (see p. 80)
3. The solubility of oxygen in the blood (small effect).

CO_2 is carried in the blood in three forms (Fig. 4.2):

1. ~90% as bicarbonate
2. ~5% in the form of carbamino compounds (CO_2 combines with the amino groups of plasma proteins and haemoglobin)
3. ~5% in physical solution (CO_2 is over 20 times more soluble in blood than is O_2).

The large bicarbonate stores of CO_2 are an important pH buffer within the blood. CO_2 levels are tightly regulated by changes in ventilation.

Fig. 4.1 Scanning electron micrograph of red blood cells showing their characteristic discoid, biconcave shape (courtesy Dr Trevor Gray). Taken with permission from A Stevens and J Lowe. Human Histology, 2nd edition. Mosby, 1997.

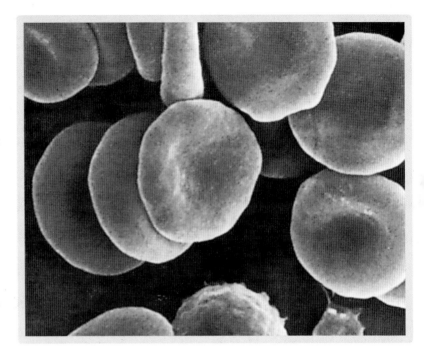

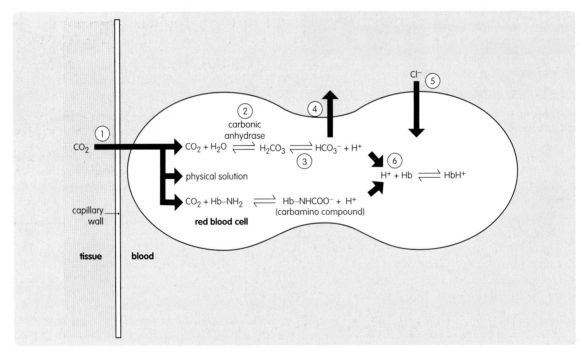

Fig. 4.2 Carbon dioxide (CO_2) transport. CO_2 is transported in both red blood cells and the plasma. Only the intracellular pathways are shown. (1) CO_2 moves along a concentration gradient from tissue to blood. (2) Carbonic anhydrase (not present in plasma) catalyses the formation of carbonic acid (H_2CO_3) from H_2O and CO_2. (3) H_2CO_3 dissociates into protons (H^+) and bicarbonate ions (HCO_3^-). (4) HCO_3^- diffuses along a concentration gradient into the plasma. (5) Chloride ions (Cl^-) enter the cell to maintain electroneutrality, a process known as the 'chloride shift'. (6) H^+, produced as a result of the dissociation of H_2CO_3 and carbamino compounds, is not able to leave the cell. Imidazole groups on the haemoglobin molecule buffer the protons.

Electrolyte balance

Chloride, potassium and hydrogen ions are transported across the red-cell membrane. One consequence of this is that, in blood stored for transfusion, the extracellular potassium level is quite high due to disruption of active transport. In large transfusions there is potential for hyperkalaemia in some cases.

ERYTHROPOIESIS

Erythropoiesis (Fig. 4.3) is the production of red blood cells from the BFU-GEMM (granulocyte, erythrocyte, monocyte, megakaryocyte) progenitor.

Sequence of erythropoiesis

Erythropoiesis occurs in erythroblastic islands within the bone marrow. These contain macrophages, which supply iron to the surrounding erythroid progenitor cells. The entire sequence (from stem cell to erythrocyte) takes approximately 1 week. Maturation is characterized by the following stages:

- Pronormoblast
- Early, intermediate and late normoblasts
- Reticulocyte
- Erythrocyte.

The production of new blood cells balances the removal of mature cells by the spleen. Following severe erythrocyte depletion, e.g. due to haemolysis, the rate of erythropoiesis in the bone marrow increases. Nucleated precursors and an increased number of reticulocytes will also appear in the peripheral blood.

Ineffective erythropoiesis

Each pronormoblast can potentially give rise to 16 erythrocytes, but some normoblasts fail to develop and are phagocytosed by bone marrow macrophages. In a healthy individual, the amount of this 'ineffective erythropoiesis' is small.

Regulation of erythropoiesis

The principal factor regulating erythropoiesis is a hormone called erythropoietin.

Erythropoietin (EPO)

EPO is a heavily glycosylated polypeptide. It is 165 amino acids in length and weighs ~30,400 kDa. It is secreted by:

Pronormoblast	The earliest erythroid cell in the bone marrow: • is large • has a small amount of basophilic (blue) cytoplasm • has a large nucleus with finely dispersed nuclear chromatin • contains lots of organelles • does not contain haemoglobin	
Early, intermediate, and late normoblasts	These cells display progressive changes in cell appearance: • decrease in cell size • decrease in nuclear size • increased condensation of chromatin • increase in cytoplasmic volume:nuclear volume ratio • decrease in blue-staining ribosomal RNA • increase in haemoglobin (stains pink) synthesis	
Reticulocyte	Reticulocytes: • are anucleate (nucleus is extruded) • contain some organelles, including ribosomes • synthesize 20–30% of total haemoglobin • are released from the bone marrow • mature after 1–2 days in peripheral blood • account for 1–2% of the red cell count • are distinguished from mature erythrocytes by brilliant cresyl blue staining (precipitated RNA appears blue)	
Erythrocyte	The mature erythrocyte appears pink and contains no organelles	

Fig. 4.3 Red cell precursors and the sequence of erythropoiesis. The appearance is that seen with the routine Romanowsky stain, unless otherwise specified.

- Endothelial cells of the peritubular capillaries in the renal cortex (90%)
- Kupffer cells and hepatocytes in the liver (10%).

Control of erythropoietin drive

The major stimulus for secretion is hypoxia. This can be caused by any factor that gives rise to decreased oxygen transport to tissues relative to tissue demand (Fig. 4.4).

Chronic renal disease (decrease in, or a complete loss of, renal mass) or bilateral nephrectomy will lead to decreased production of EPO, resulting in anaemia. Renal cell carcinomas can produce excess EPO, resulting in an erythrocytosis.

Recombinant EPO, produced in animal cells, may currently be used for:

- Anaemia due to renal failure
- Autologous blood transfusions
- After chemotherapy or bone marrow transplantation
- Anaemia of chronic disease.

In the UK the use of recombinant EPO is currently limited by the availability of funding.

Erythropoiesis is also regulated by the availability of red cell nutrients, most importantly iron, folic acid and vitamin B_{12}.

IRON AND HAEM METABOLISM

Iron metabolism

Uptake and excretion of iron

Normal uptake and excretion of iron is illustrated in Fig. 4.5. The total iron store of the body is around 4 g, mainly as haemoglobin (Fig. 4.6). The daily requirement is normally around 1 mg. Absorption is controlled by proteins in the gut. The rate of iron transfer from epithelial cells to plasma responds to iron requirements, e.g. it is high when stores are low or the rate of erythropoiesis is high.

Iron transport proteins

Free iron is toxic and is therefore incorporated into haem or bound to protein within the body.

Fig. 4.4 Regulation of erythropoietin (EPO) production. Reduced oxygen (O_2) supply to renal sensors stimulates EPO production. If this is chronically activated, extramedullary erythropoiesis can occur.

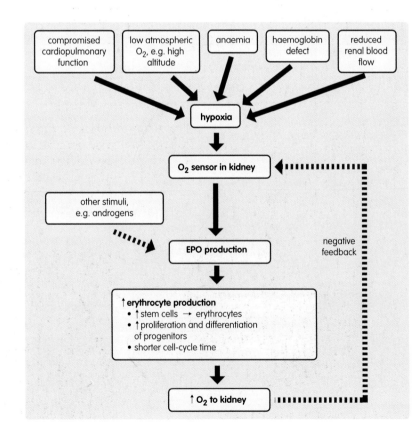

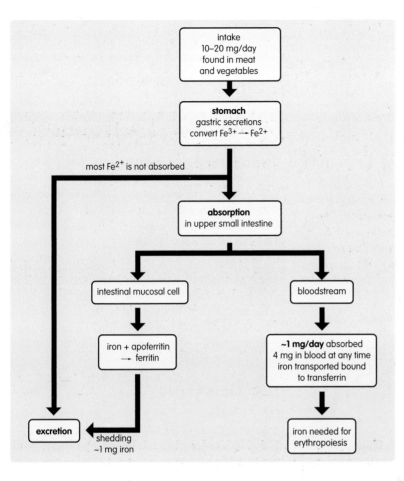

Fig. 4.5 Uptake and excretion of iron. Iron is converted in the stomach from Fe^{3+} to Fe^{2+}. This process is promoted by ascorbic acid and other reducing agents and inhibited by phytates, tannic acid and tetracycline. The ferrous form, Fe^{2+}, is actively absorbed in the duodenum and jejunum. Within intestinal mucosal cells, some iron binds apoferritin to form ferritin, a storage compound. The rest is transported, by transferrin in the blood, to storage compartments and the bone marrow. A total of 1 mg of iron is absorbed into the bloodstream each day. Total daily iron turnover is ~25 mg. Iron in shed mucosal cells or not absorbed from the diet is excreted in the faeces, although a small amount is lost from shed skin cells and excreted in the urine. Extra iron is lost during menstruation (1.5 mg per day compared with 1 mg normally).

Transferrin transports up to two molecules of iron to tissues that have transferrin receptors, e.g. bone marrow. Ferritin is a water-soluble compound, consisting of protein and iron. Haemosiderin is insoluble and consists of aggregates of ferritin that have partially lost their protein component.

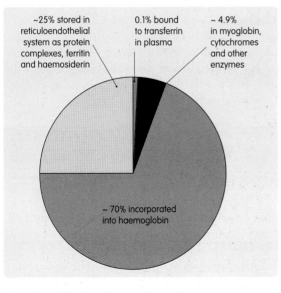

Fig. 4.6 Distribution of iron in the body.

Iron is found in green vegetables and meats in ferric–protein and haem–protein complexes, respectively. Ferric iron is poorly absorbed compared to haem, thus putting vegetarians and vegans at an increased risk of iron deficiency. Consumption of vitamin C with a source of ferric iron aids its absorption, as vitamin C forms complexes with and reduces the ferric iron to ferrous.

Iron overload

There is no mechanism for the excretion of excess iron. Consequently, iron overload can occur as a result of:

- Increased absorption
- Parenteral administration.

Increased absorption

This can be either primary or secondary, and results from the following:

- Primary/hereditary haemochromatosis—an autosomal recessive disorder characterized by excessive intestinal absorption of iron
- Erythroid hyperplasia secondary to ineffective erythropoiesis or haemolysis, e.g. thalassaemia syndromes
- Dietary excess (rare)
- Inappropriate oral therapy.

> **Haemochromatosis**
>
> This condition is autosomal recessive. The gene mutation HFE is located on chromosome 6 and codes for a transmembrane protein that modulates iron uptake. Heterozygotes are at an increased risk of secondary forms of haemosiderosis if they have other risk factors.
>
> Clinical features of presentation after the age of 40 include hepatomegaly (which may progress to cirrhosis), bronze skin pigmentation, chondrocalcinosis, pseudogout, diabetes mellitus, hypopituitarism, hypogonadism, cardiac arrhythmias and cardiomyopathy.
>
> Management includes screening first degree relatives, venesection, chelation with desferrioxamine and liver transplant.

> Secondary forms of iron overload are called haemosiderosis.

Parenteral administration

- Multiple blood transfusions (1 unit of blood contains ~250 mg of iron)
- Inappropriate parenteral iron therapy.

Treatment

It is important to start therapy as soon as possible to prevent irreversible organ damage. Options include:

- Dietary advice (decrease intake of iron, increase intake of natural chelators)
- Venesection
- Chelation therapy—desferrioxamine is an iron-chelating agent that is administered subcutaneously or intravenously. There is now a new oral iron chelating agent, deferiprone, licensed for the treatment of iron overload in thalassaemia.

Haem metabolism

Haem belongs to a family of compounds known as the porphyrins, which are characterized by the presence of a tetrapyrrole ring. Haem is an iron-containing derivative, the iron atom being located at the centre of the tetrapyrrole ring of protoporphyrin IX. The haem group is responsible for the oxygen-binding properties of haemoglobin.

Haem biosynthesis

Haem synthesis occurs in the mitochondria by a process outlined in Fig. 4.7.

Haem breakdown

Degradation occurs in the macrophages of the spleen, bone marrow and liver (Fig. 4.8). In haemolytic anaemias, red cells have a shortened lifespan because they are destroyed at an accelerated rate. This increased red-cell destruction leads to anaemia, which stimulates increased EPO production, leading to compensatory erythropoiesis. The clinical features of haemolytic anaemias result from the increased red-cell destruction and the compensatory increase in red-cell production (Fig. 4.9).

HAEMOGLOBIN

Structure of haemoglobin

Haemoglobin is composed of four globin chains held together by non-covalent interactions (Fig. 4.10). Each chain is associated with a prosthetic haem group, the oxygen-binding site of the molecule. Each globin chain has a hydrophobic crevice, or haem pocket, which contains the haem molecule. Proximal histidine molecules bind to the iron

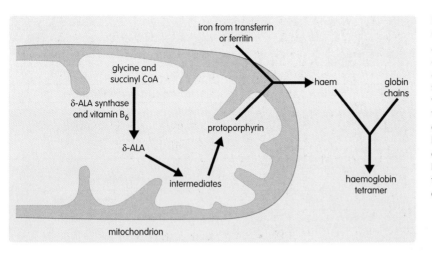

Fig. 4.7 Haem biosynthesis. Glycine and succinyl coenzyme A (CoA) combine to form δ-aminolaevulinic acid (δ-ALA), a reaction controlled by δ-ALA synthase and the coenzyme vitamin B_6. δ-ALA is converted to protoporphyrin, which combines ferrous iron to form haem. The haem molecule combines with a globin chain. Haemoglobin is formed by a tetramer of these haem–globin complexes.

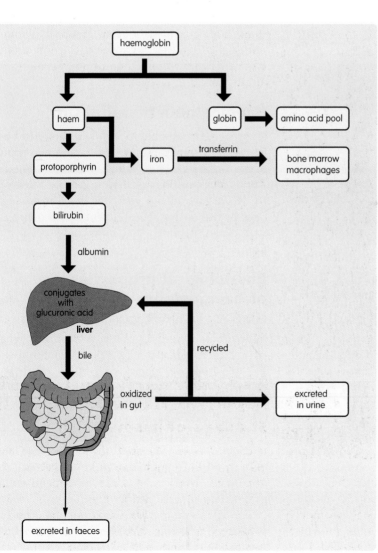

Fig. 4.8 Degradation of haemoglobin. Amino acids from the globin chains are recycled to produce new proteins. Iron is transported by transferrin to the bone marrow to produce new erythrocytes. Protoporphyrin is degraded to bilirubin, which is conjugated by the liver and excreted in bile. Bilirubin is excreted in the faeces or converted to urobilinogen, reabsorbed and excreted in the urine.

Fig. 4.9 Clinical features of haemolytic anaemias

Cause	Clinical feature	Mechanism
Increased red-cell destruction	Pallor of mucous membranes	↓ Haemoglobin
	Jaundice	↑ Unconjugated serum bilirubin
	Urine darkens on standing	↑ Urobilinogen
	Pigment gallstones	↑ Bilirubin in bile
	Splenomegaly	↑ Red cell destruction
	Absence of plasma haptoglobins	Hb binds haptoglobins; this complex is then removed by macrophages
	Reticulocytosis	Erythrocyte precursors enter the blood
Increased red-cell production	Folate deficiency	Increased erythropoiesis
	Bone deformities	Erythroid hyperplasia causes expansion of marrow cavities

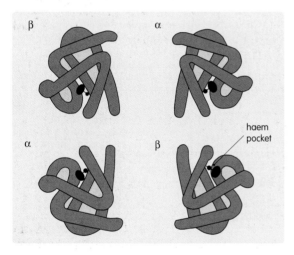

Fig. 4.10 Structure of adult haemoglobin. The α-chain is 141 amino acids long; the β-chain 146 amino acids. A haem pocket can be seen in each globin chain.

portion of the haem molecule, and distal histidine molecules help stabilize iron in its ferrous state. The haem pocket allows O_2 binding, while protecting the iron atom from oxidation.

Different types of haemoglobin are present at different stages of development (Fig. 4.11). Adult haemoglobin (HbA) contains two α- and two β-chains, which are arranged as two dimers, written $2(\alpha\beta)$. The globin chains interact with each other in an allosteric fashion. Binding of one O_2 increases the affinity for oxygen at the remaining haem groups.

The other major haem-containing protein in humans is myoglobin, which consists of a single chain associated with a haem group. It is found principally in muscle, where it provides an oxygen reserve. The four haemoglobin subunits are structurally similar to myoglobin.

Haemoglobin metabolism

The genes encoding the ε-, γ-, δ- and β-chains are found on chromosome 11. The ζ- and two copies of the α-chain genes are found on chromosome 16. The relative positions of these genes are shown in Fig. 4.12. Each globin gene has three exons separated by two introns. The different globin chains are synthesized separately and then come together to form a functional Hb molecule.

Physiological properties of haemoglobin

Each haemoglobin molecule (Hb) can bind four molecules of oxygen, one at each haem site. When Hb is oxygenated, relaxed (R-) Hb, the globin chains are able to move against each other, which will allow O_2 release. When O_2 is unloaded, the metabolite 2,3-diphosphoglycerate (2,3-DPG) enters the centre of the deoxyhaemoglobin molecule, reducing its affinity for O_2. Deoxyhaemoglobin, taut (T-) haemoglobin, is characterized by a relatively large number of ionic and hydrogen bonds between the αβ dimers, which restrict the movement of the globin chains.

The oxygen dissociation curve is a plot of partial pressure of oxygen (x axis) against oxygen saturation (y axis) (Fig. 4.13).

Fig. 4.11 Types of haemoglobin present during different stages of development

Developmental stage	Haemoglobin type	Chains	Note
Embryonic	Hb Gower I Hb Gower II Hb Portland	$\zeta_2\varepsilon_2$ $\alpha_2\varepsilon_2$ $\zeta_2\gamma_2$	
Fetal	HbF	$\alpha_2\gamma_2$	Main Hb in later two-thirds of fetal life and in the newborn; higher affinity for O_2 than HbA
Adult	HbA HbA$_2$	$\alpha_2\beta_2$ $\alpha_2\delta_2$	Principal Hb; 68,000 kDa ~2% of adult Hb

Hb, haemoglobin; HbA, adult haemoglobin; HbF, fetal haemoglobin.

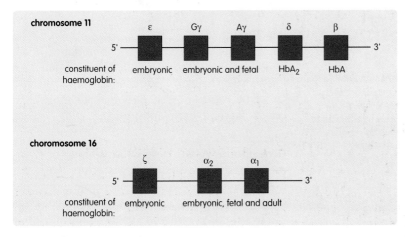

Fig. 4.12 The relative positions of the globin genes. The genes are arranged in the order in which they are expressed during development. The Gγ and Aγ genes encode γ-chains that differ by just one amino acid. HbA, adult haemoglobin.

The shift of the oxygen dissociation curve to the right in the presence of increased H^+ concentration is called the Bohr effect. This is not the cause of increased ventilatory rate, which is driven by trying to lower CO_2.

Changes in CO_2, H^+, 2,3-DPG and temperature shift the position of the haemoglobin curve but do not generally alter its shape (Fig. 4.13). H^+ and 2,3-DPG bind to and stabilize deoxyhaemoglobin, favouring the unloading of oxygen. Oxygen binding to myoglobin is not altered by these factors. Haemoglobin variants also have an effect on the oxygen dissociation curve, e.g. sickle-cell haemoglobin shifts the curve to the right. If the curve is shifted to the right, a normal exercise tolerance can be achieved, even with a low haemoglobin count.

High concentrations of 2,3-DPG are present in red cells. During periods of hypoxia, levels of 2,3-DPG are increased, increasing oxygen release in the tissues. Oxygen is transferred from adult to fetal haemoglobin (HbF) because 2,3-DPG binds to HbF less effectively than to adult Hb (HbA). In blood stored in acid–citrate–dextrose, red-cell 2,3-DPG levels decline, causing an abnormally high affinity for oxygen and resulting in poor unloading in the tissues.

THE CYTOSKELETON OF THE RED CELL

Structure

The erythrocyte plasma membrane is supported by a dense, fibrillar, protein shell—the cytoskeleton.

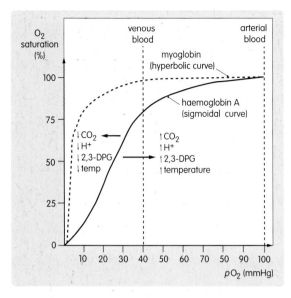

Fig. 4.13 Oxygen dissociation curve for haemoglobin and myoglobin. The haemoglobin curve is sigmoidal in shape because of the cooperative binding of O_2 to haemoglobin. Conversely, unloading of O_2 at one haem group facilitates unloading at the other haem sites. In comparison, the myoglobin curve is hyperbolic in shape, because myoglobin does not release oxygen until the partial pressure of O_2 (pO_2) falls to very low levels. This is because myoglobin does not exhibit cooperative binding. HbA is 100% saturated at a pO_2 of 100 mmHg and 75% saturated at 40 mmHg, the partial pressures of arterial and venous blood, respectively. 2,3-DPG, 2,3-diphosphoglycerate.

The red-cell cytoskeleton:

- Maintains cell shape and confers strength to the erythrocyte membrane, allowing the cell to withstand the stresses of the circulation
- Permits flexibility, which is important in erythrocyte circulation.

The proteins of the plasma membrane, both integral and peripheral, are important constituents of the cytoskeleton (Fig. 4.14). The band numbers refer to their mobility on electrophoresis.

Integral proteins

Integral proteins penetrate the lipid bilayer and are closely associated with it.

Band 3 protein

Band 3 protein is a glycoprotein homodimer, which transports anions (Cl^-, HCO_3^-). It has binding sites for ankyrin, band 4.1 protein, haemoglobin and glycolytic enzymes. The carbohydrate moiety expresses Ii blood group antigens.

Glycophorins

Glycophorins A, B, C and D are a group of glycoproteins with the same gross structure. Each has three domains: receptor, transmembranous and cytoplasmic.

The cytoplasmic domain of glycophorin A binds cytoskeletal proteins. The receptor domain of glycophorin A has receptors for lectins and influenza virus. Glycophorin A expresses MN blood group antigens; glycophorin B expresses N, Ss and U blood group antigens.

Fig. 4.14 Structure of the red cell cytoskeleton. The hexagonal spectrin lattice is anchored to the membrane by band 3 protein, ankyrin and band 4.1 protein.

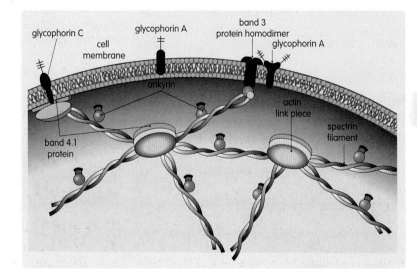

Peripheral proteins

Peripheral proteins are loosely attached to the lipid bilayer.

Spectrin (bands 1 and 2)

Spectrin is the primary structural component of the cytoskeleton. The α and β subunits of spectrin twist around each other to form heterodimers, which associate to produce tetramers. Tetramers of spectrin are bound together by interactions with band 4.1 protein and actin to form a hexagonal lattice.

Ankyrin

Ankyrin consists of bands 2.1–2.3 and 2.6. It has binding sites for the β-chain of spectrin and band 3 protein.

Band 4.1 protein

Band 4.1 protein binds spectrin, strengthening the lattice structure. It also binds band 3 protein and glycophorin.

Actin

Actin, also known as band 5, is present in the F actin configuration (short filaments). It binds α- and β-spectrin, supporting the lattice of spectrin tetramers.

The cytoskeleton in disease

Hereditary spherocytosis

This is an autosomal dominant haemolytic anaemia caused by deficiency or dysfunction of one of the skeletal proteins of the erythrocyte membrane, resulting in poorly deformable erythrocytes which appear spherical down the microscope. The protein most commonly implicated is spectrin (Fig. 4.15). The disordered cytoskeleton network accelerates red-cell destruction, as long as the patient has a spleen.

METABOLISM OF RED CELLS

Glucose is the principal energy source for red cells. It is taken up by facilitated diffusion in an insulin-independent fashion. Because red cells have no mitochondria they cannot metabolize glucose aerobically, therefore it is metabolized via:

- The glycolytic pathway (Embden–Meyerhof pathway)
- The hexose monophosphate shunt.

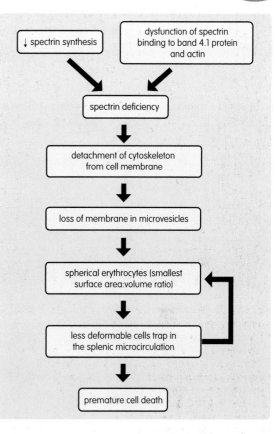

Fig. 4.15 Mechanism of spherocytosis and premature cell death in hereditary spherocytosis due to spectrin deficiency.

Glycolysis and the Embden–Meyerhof pathway

This is the glycolytic pathway common to all cells of the human body whereby glucose is metabolized to lactate (Fig. 4.16). There is a net yield of two ATP molecules, but no net NADH production.

$$\text{glucose} + 2P_i + 2ADP \rightarrow 2 \text{ lactate} + 2ATP + 2H_2O$$

Defects of glycolytic enzymes are rare. Approximately 95% are associated with pyruvate kinase and are restricted to red blood cells. Insufficient ATP is produced to maintain the structural integrity of the red cell, leading to premature cell death and a haemolytic anaemia.

The Luebering–Rapoport shunt

This branch of the glycolytic pathway generates 2,3-diphosphoglycerate (2,3-DPG), as illustrated in

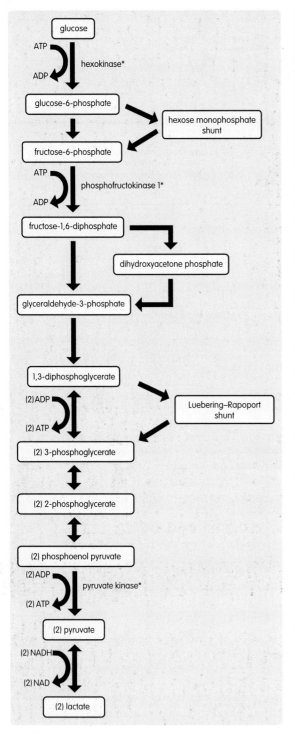

Fig. 4.16 The Embden–Meyerhof pathway. Starred enzymes represent the rate-limiting steps. ADP, adenosine diphosphate; ATP, adenosine triphosphate; NAD/NADH, nicotinamide adenine dinucleotide.

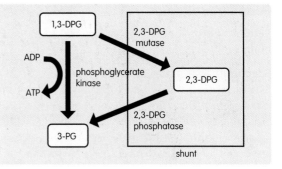

Fig. 4.17 The Luebering–Rapoport shunt. The reaction shown occurs twice per glucose molecule. DPG, diphosphoglycerate; PG, phosphoglycerate.

Fig. 4.17. Trace amounts of 2,3-DPG are found in most cells but high concentrations are found in red cells, where it is important in regulating the affinity of haemoglobin for oxygen. Between 15% and 25% of glucose passing through the glycolytic pathway enters this shunt. In doing so, the reaction catalysed by phosphoglycerate kinase is bypassed, and no net ATP is produced.

The hexose monophosphate shunt

This is also known as the pentose phosphate pathway. Under normal conditions, 5% of the glucose metabolized by the red cell passes through an oxidative pathway of metabolism, the hexose monophosphate (HMP) shunt (Fig. 4.18). There is no net ATP yield, but two NADPH molecules are produced per molecule of glucose-6-phosphate entering the shunt. The majority of the cell's NADPH is produced in this way. NADPH is important in erythrocytes because it reduces oxidized glutathione (GSSG). Reduced glutathione (GSH) is required to maintain sulphydryl groups in their reduced state, which maintains the integrity of haemoglobin and the cytoskeleton.

Glucose-6-phosphate dehydrogenase deficiency is an X-linked disorder characterized by a lack of the enzyme or by a dysfunctional enzyme. Patients are usually asymptomatic, but oxidant stress can induce acute episodes of haemolysis (Fig. 4.19).

Prevention of haem oxidation

When haemoglobin is oxidized ($Fe^{2+} \rightarrow Fe^{3+}$) it is known as methaemoglobin (metHb). Excess metHb is caused by:

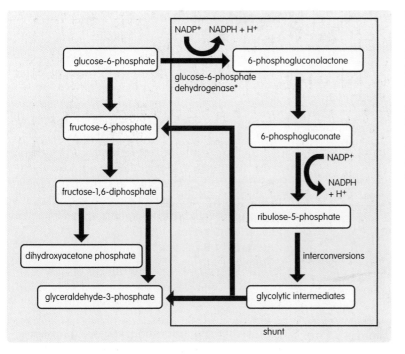

Fig. 4.18 The hexose monophosphate shunt. The first three reactions constitute the irreversible oxidative portion of the pathway and are the sites of NADPH production. The remainder of the pathway is non-oxidative and, in addition to glycolytic intermediates, produces ribulose-5-phosphate, which is used for nucleotide synthesis. The starred enzyme represents the rate-limiting step.

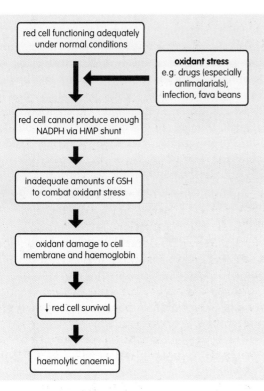

Fig. 4.19 Mechanism of haemolysis in glucose-6-phosphate dehydrogenase deficiency. GSH, reduced glutathione; HMP, hexose monophosphate; NADPH, nicotinamide adenine dinucleotide phosphate.

- Toxic substances
- Abnormal haemoglobins resistant to enzymatic reduction (M haemoglobins)
- NADH methaemoglobin reductase deficiency (rare).

The reduced haemoglobin can bind to albumin and has a reduced oxygen-carrying capability. NADH from the Embden–Meyerhof pathway and NADH methaemoglobin reductase are important in ensuring that iron remains in its reduced form.

ANAEMIA

Anaemia is a low level of haemoglobin in the blood. Haemoglobin values less than 13 g/dL for men and 12 g/dL for women indicate anaemia, although this does not indicate the need for a blood transfusion.

Anaemia is a common problem worldwide, affecting as much as a third of the world's population. It can be caused by decreased production or increased destruction of erythrocytes, or by blood loss. In developing countries, dietary deficiency and blood loss due to parasitic gut infections are common. In the UK, decreased production is the most common cause.

The physiological response to anaemia attempts to maintain adequate oxygenation of the body. The level of 2,3-DPG rises to ensure that oxygen is unloaded at the tissues. The cardiac output increases and the circulation becomes hyperdynamic. This can be detected by a rapid pulse and heart murmurs. Anaemic patients are often pale. Symptoms vary depending on the cause, but include:

- Fatigue
- Dyspnoea
- Palpitations
- Headache
- Tinnitus
- Anorexia and bowel disturbance.

Anaemias may be classified either morphologically or by cause. Anaemias are micro-, normo- or macrocytic, depending on the mean cell volume (MCV). The mean amount of haemoglobin in each erythrocyte (MCH) is also measured. If the MCH is low, the anaemia is hypochromic.

ANAEMIA DUE TO IMPAIRED RED-CELL PRODUCTION

Megaloblastic anaemias

In megaloblastic anaemias, impaired DNA synthesis results in the appearance of megaloblasts (abnormal red cell precursors) in the marrow. Megaloblasts are large cells which contain relatively large abnormal nuclei with finely dispersed chromatin. Anaemia occurs because megaloblasts are removed by bone marrow phagocytes (ineffective erythropoiesis). Megaloblastic anaemia is usually due to deficiency of vitamin B_{12} and/or folate. Both act as coenzymes in the pathway of DNA synthesis. Haematological findings include:

- Macrocytic anaemia (leucopenia and thrombocytopenia in severe megaloblastic anaemia)
- Hypersegmentation of neutrophil nuclei
- Megaloblasts seen on bone marrow smear
- Low serum vitamin B_{12} levels or reduced red cell folate content.

Vitamin B_{12} deficiency

Vitamin B_{12} consists of cobalamin bound to a methyl or adenosyl group. It is found only in foods of animal origin and is not affected by cooking. Absorption occurs in the terminal ileum after combining with intrinsic factor (IF) secreted from gastric parietal cells. Transport within the body is with the plasma-binding protein transcobalamin II.

Vitamin B_{12} is stored in the liver. Body stores are large (~2–3 mg), and the daily rate of loss in urine and faeces is small relative to daily requirements (1–2 μg); therefore it takes more than 2 years after the onset of the cause of vitamin B_{12} deficiency for anaemia to develop.

Causes of B_{12} deficiency include:

- Dietary, e.g. due to veganism (rare)
- Intrinsic factor deficiency, e.g. due to pernicious anaemia, postgastrectomy or congenital
- Intestinal malabsorption, e.g. due to diseases of the terminal ileum, such as Crohn's disease
- Blind loop or diverticulae in the small bowel which breed bacteria that utilize vitamin B_{12}.

Pernicious anaemia

Pernicious anaemia is an autoimmune chronic atrophic gastritis and is the most common cause of vitamin B_{12} deficiency in adults. Autoantibodies directed against both the gastric parietal cells and IF are detectable in the serum and gastric juice of most patients. Damage to the parietal cells results in failure of IF secretion and vitamin B_{12} absorption. Achlorhydria is an accompanying feature (parietal cells are also responsible for secreting H^+). Pernicious anaemia is associated with autoimmune thyroid disease and patients are at increased risk of gastric carcinoma.

Clinical features of vitamin B_{12} deficiency include:

- A lemon-yellow colour to the skin (if severe), due to a combination of pallor and jaundice
- Glossitis
- Gastrointestinal disturbances
- Weight loss
- Neurological abnormalities (peripheral neuropathy, subacute degeneration of the cord involving the posterior and lateral columns)
- Psychiatric disturbances.

The Schilling test is used to diagnose the cause of vitamin B_{12} deficiency, the steps of which are as follows:

1. Oral, radioactively labelled vitamin B_{12} and intramuscular, non-radioactive vitamin B_{12} are administered simultaneously. The intramuscular B_{12} saturates the B_{12}-binding proteins in the plasma, promoting urinary excretion of any absorbed radioactive B_{12}
2. The urine is collected for 24 hours after B_{12} administration. If less than 10% of the orally administered B_{12} is excreted, absorption of B_{12} is considered impaired
3. The test is repeated, but this time both oral IF and oral B_{12} are given. If impaired absorption is due to lack of IF (as in pernicious anaemia), B_{12} absorption will be increased. B_{12} absorption will not be increased if the cause of deficiency is malabsorption.

Treatment of vitamin B_{12} deficiency is by correction of the underlying cause, if possible, and intramuscular injections of vitamin B_{12} approximately every 3 months.

Folate deficiency

Folates are derived from folic (pteroyl glutamic) acid. They are found in foods, mainly green vegetables and liver, and are destroyed by cooking. Absorption takes place in the duodenum and jejunum. Folate is stored in the liver. Unlike vitamin B_{12}, folate stores are small (10–15 mg) and daily losses are larger relative to daily requirement (100–200 µg), therefore a megaloblastic anaemia develops a few months after the onset of folate deficiency.

Causes of folate deficiency are:

- Decreased intake, e.g. due to poor diet
- Decreased absorption, e.g. due to coeliac disease
- Increased requirement due to rapid cell multiplication, e.g. caused by pregnancy, prematurity, malignancy or haemolytic anaemia
- Increased loss, e.g. due to dialysis
- Drugs, e.g. ethanol, methotrexate (by inhibition of dihydrofolate reductase), trimethoprim, anticonvulsants and possibly the oral contraceptive pill.

Alcohol causes folate deficiency because of malabsorption, malnutrition and increased utilization.

Clinical features of folate deficiency are similar to those of vitamin B_{12} deficiency, without the neurological and psychiatric abnormalities. Treatment of folate deficiency is by correction of any underlying cause and oral supplements of folic acid. If there is a possibility of vitamin B_{12} deficiency, supplements should be given at the same time as folic acid to prevent neurological complications.

Red cell folate is low in both vitamin B_{12} and folate deficiency. A serum folate should be used to differentiate between the two.

Iron-deficiency anaemia

Iron deficiency is the most common cause of anaemia worldwide. It occurs most frequently in women of reproductive age. Anaemia occurs after iron stores have been depleted. Causes of iron-deficiency anaemia include:

- Decreased iron intake, e.g. due to poor diet
- Increased iron requirement, e.g. during growth, pregnancy and lactation
- Chronic blood loss, e.g. due to peptic ulcer
- Decreased iron absorption, e.g. after gastrectomy.

The signs and symptoms of iron-deficiency anaemia (Fig. 4.20) are often only apparent when the haemoglobin level drops below 8 g/dL. The haematological findings are:

- A microcytic, hypochromic anaemia
- Reduced serum iron and ferritin (to distinguish from thalassaemia syndromes)
- Increased serum transferrin and total iron-binding capacity (TIBC) (to distinguish from anaemia of chronic disease)
- Reduced plasma transferrin saturation
- Absence of iron stores demonstrated on bone-marrow smear.

Treatment is by oral administration of iron in the form of ferrous sulphate tablets. This must be continued for 4–6 months to replenish iron stores. Any underlying cause should be treated. Parenteral iron is used if the patient has malabsorption or cannot tolerate oral preparations.

Fig. 4.20 Signs and symptoms of iron-deficiency anaemia

Features common to other anaemias	Features specific to iron deficiency
• Fatigue • Dizziness • Headache • Shortness of breath • Palpitations • Angina • Intermittent claudication • Pallor • Tachycardia • Flow murmur • Congestive cardiac failure	• Glossitis (smooth, sore, red tongue) • Koilonychia (spoon-shaped nails) • Angular stomatitis (sores and cracks at corners of mouth) • Alopecia • Pica (unusual dietary cravings, e.g. for clay and ice)

An atrophic gastritis can also be seen with iron deficiency. In Plummer–Vinson or Paterson–Kelly syndrome, dysphagia and pharyngeal or oesophageal webs accompany the iron-deficiency anaemia.

Other causes of microcytic anaemia that should be considered are:

- Sideroblastic anaemia (hereditary and acquired). Some respond to vitamin B_6, particularly the former. Vitamin B_6 is a cofactor for haem synthesis, and deficiency prevents iron incorporation. Ringed sideroblasts, red-cell precursors containing iron granules surrounding the nucleus, are seen in the bone marrow (see also p. 78).
- Lead poisoning, which also causes abdominal pain and neuropathy.

ANAEMIA DUE TO INCREASED RED-CELL DESTRUCTION (HAEMOLYTIC ANAEMIAS)

Haemolytic anaemias occur when red cell lifespan is reduced. Erythropoiesis can normally be increased seven-fold, therefore haemolysis may be compensated and not cause anaemia. Reduced red cell lifespan can be caused by erythrocyte defects or extracorpuscular defects, as shown in Fig. 4.21. It can occur within the circulation or be extravascular:

- **Extravascular haemolysis:** is the route by which red cells are normally broken down and occurs in the macrophages of the spleen, bone marrow and liver
- **Intravascular haemolysis:** is the destruction of red cells within the circulation. It is characterized by all of the features of extravascular haemolysis (see Fig. 4.9, p. 80), as well as by the following:
  - haemoglobinaemia: Hb is released into the bloodstream
  - absence of plasma haptoglobins: Hb binds haptoglobin to form a complex that is removed by macrophages in the reticuloendothelial system
  - haemoglobinuria: the Hb concentration exceeds the tubular reabsorptive capacity and Hb is therefore excreted in the urine
  - haemosiderinuria: proximal tubule cells containing intracellular deposits of haemosiderin derived from the Hb reabsorbed in the kidneys are shed in the urine
  - methaemalbuminaemia: some of the Hb is oxidized and binds to albumin
  - reticulocytosis: erythrocyte precursors enter the blood (also found in extravascular haemolysis).

Fig. 4.21 Classification of haemolytic anaemias

Erythrocyte defects		Extracorpuscular defects	
Membrane	Hereditary spherocytosis Hereditary elliptocytosis Paroxysmal nocturnal haemoglobinuria	Immune	Incompatible transfusions Autoimmune haemolytic anaemia Drug associated
Enzyme	G6PD deficiency PK deficiency	Infection	Malaria Septicaemia
Haemoglobin	Sickle-cell syndromes Thalassaemia	Drugs/chemicals	Dapsone, sulfasalazine
		Mechanical	Microangiopathic haemolysis Prosthetic heart valves DIC, HUS, TTP Following long marches
		Hypersplenism	Myelofibrosis

DIC, disseminated intravascular coagulation; G6PD, glucose-6-phosphate dehydrogenase; HUS, haemolytic uraemic syndrome; PK, pyruvate kinase; TTP, thrombotic thrombocytopenic purpura.

Hereditary red-cell defects

The defect is usually intrinsic to the red cell, and morphological abnormalities can often be detected on inspection of a peripheral blood smear.

Cytoskeleton defects

Hereditary spherocytosis

Hereditary spherocytosis is a common (prevalence of 1 in 5000 in northern Europe) autosomal dominant disorder of variable penetrance. A defective cytoskeletal protein, most commonly spectrin, causes loss of the membrane. This results in progressive spherocytosis and reduced deformability of red cells, leading to extravascular haemolysis (see Fig. 4.15, p. 83). Haematological findings include:

- Spherocytes on the peripheral blood smear
- Increased osmotic fragility: when suspended in saline solutions of varying concentrations, spherocytes lyse in less hypotonic solutions than do normal red cells.

The person can be asymptomatic or haemolysis can be present at birth with significant jaundice and anaemia. The usual course after infancy is a low-grade anaemia with intermittent 'crises'. Splenectomy can be used to prevent crises and will result in a rise in the Hb level. Pneumococcal, meningococcal and Hib vaccines should be administered before the operation and prophylactic penicillin is recommended postoperatively.

Hereditary elliptocytosis

This autosomal dominant disorder is also due to abnormalities of the cytoskeletal proteins and is most commonly caused by failure of spectrin dimers to form tetramers. It is clinically similar to, but milder than, hereditary spherocytosis. A high proportion of elliptical red cells are seen on the peripheral blood film.

Enzyme defects

Pyruvate kinase deficiency

This is a rare autosomal recessive condition affecting the glycolytic pathway, which results in a lack of ATP production. Erythrocytes become rigid and are destroyed. The blood film shows a poikilocytosis and distorted 'prickle' cells (seen postsplenectomy). Splenectomy might improve, but not cure, the anaemia.

Glucose-6-phosphate dehydrogenase deficiency

Glucose-6-phosphate dehydrogenase (G6PD) deficiency is an X-linked disorder affecting the hexose monophosphate shunt. There are over 400 variants of G6PD, two of which account for the vast majority of cases: the African and Mediterranean types. Of these two, the Mediterranean type is clinically more severe, because of a much greater reduction in enzyme function. Patients are generally asymptomatic until haemolysis is precipitated by oxidizing factors such as:

- Infection
- Acidosis, e.g. diabetic ketoacidosis
- Drugs, e.g. primaquine, sulphonamides
- Fava beans ('favism'—only in the Mediterranean type).

Haemolysis is primarily intravascular. During a haemolytic crisis, Heinz bodies (precipitates of oxidized, denatured Hb) are generated within red blood cells. Cells that have had Heinz bodies removed upon passing through the spleen, termed 'bite' or 'blister' cells, are seen on the peripheral blood film. Heinz bodies will be seen in patients following splenectomy.

In an asymptomatic patient, the peripheral blood film might be normal. However, G6PD levels are decreased in affected males and carrier females. Assay can be unreliable during or immediately after a haemolytic crisis because reticulocytes (increased in number during a crisis) have higher enzyme levels than mature red cells. In an acute crisis, the precipitating factor should be eliminated and the circulation supported; however, there is no specific treatment.

Other enzyme defects
Several other defects have been identified in enzymes involved in erythrocyte metabolism. They are rare and include hexokinase and glutathione synthetase.

Haemoglobin defects

Thalassaemias

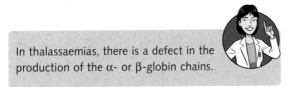

In thalassaemias, there is a defect in the production of the α- or β-globin chains.

β-Thalassaemia occurs most commonly in Mediterranean countries, South-East Asia and Africa. There is a partial or complete failure of β-globin chain production due to:

- Incorrect excision of introns from mRNA (most common)
- Mutations of the regulatory sequences
- Mutations affecting capping
- Mutations affecting polyadenylation of mRNA
- β-Chain gene mutations.

The abnormal β-chain genes are denoted $β^+$ and $β^0$ for partial or complete deficiency, respectively. Severity of disease depends on which abnormal genes have been inherited and whether the individual is heterozygous or homozygous.

α-Thalassaemia is most common in South-East Asia and West Africa. There is a deletion of one, two, three or all four α-globin chain genes. The number of deleted genes relates to the severity of disease, although deletion of all four α-globin chains is incompatible with life.

An excess of α-chains (in β-thalassaemia) or β-chains (in α-thalassaemia) results in abnormal aggregation within red-cell precursors, predisposing them to phagocytosis by bone marrow macrophages. Any abnormal red cells that reach the circulation have a shortened lifespan. A number of clinical syndromes are recognized, based on the severity of the anaemia (Fig. 4.22).

β-Thalassaemia major
In β-thalassaemia major, homozygosity for defective genes causes β-chain production to be severely reduced. Investigation reveals:

- Microcytic hypochromic anaemia (Hb 2–3 g/dL) and reticulocytosis (at 6–9 months if not transfused)
- Basophilic stippling, target cells and normoblasts on peripheral blood film
- Absence of HbA on electrophoresis
- High serum iron due to increased enteric absorption and regular blood transfusions
- A 'hair-on-end' appearance on skull X-ray (Fig. 4.23). Bony changes are caused by expansion of haemopoietic bone marrow from its normal sites.

Treatment is by regular blood transfusions (about one a month), splenectomy and/or bone marrow transplantation. Chelation therapy is given to prevent iron overload.

β-Thalassaemia minor
This is often known as β-thalassaemia trait because it is heterozygous. Patients are often asymptomatic, but will usually have microcytic red blood cells and a mild anaemia. Recognition of this syndrome is important as it has implications for genetic counselling and can also mimic iron-deficiency anaemia, for which inappropriate iron therapy might be given.

Fig. 4.22 Thalassaemia syndromes

Clinical syndrome	Type	Presentation
β-thalassaemia major (Mediterranean or Cooley's anaemia)	Homozygous ($\beta^0\beta^0$, $\beta^+\beta^+$ or $\beta^+\beta^0$)	Onset at 6–9 months; severe anaemia, jaundice, failure to thrive, hepatosplenomegaly, bony abnormalities, gallstones, leg ulcers, intercurrent infections
β-thalassaemia intermedia	A variety of genotypes	Presents at 1–2 years of age with a moderate anaemia
β-thalassaemia minor	Heterozygous ($\beta^0\beta$ or $\beta^+\beta$)	Usually asymptomatic; mild microcytic hypochromic anaemia (Hb 10–11 g/dL) Raised HbA_2 (4–8% of total Hb)
Silent carrier	3 α genes present	Usually asymptomatic with no detected abnormalities
α-thalassaemia trait	2 α genes present	Normal or slightly low haemoglobin level with microcytic red cells, usually asymptomatic
HbH disease	1 α gene present	Anaemia (7–11 g/dL); HbH is formed (β_4) Clinical features of chronic haemolysis
Hydrops fetalis	No α genes present	Fetus usually dies in utero Tetramers of γ-chains form a haemoglobin variant, Hb Barts hydrops Prenatal diagnosis with aggressive transfusions in utero can prevent fetal death

Hb, haemoglobin; HbA, adult haemoglobin; HbF, fetal haemoglobin.

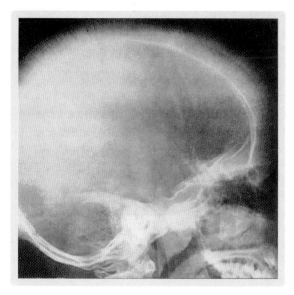

Fig. 4.23 Skull radiograph of a child with β-thalassaemia major. The 'hair-on-end' appearance is pathognomonic. It is caused by extramedullary haemopoiesis.

Sickle-cell syndromes

The sickle Hb (HbS) gene is prevalent in tropical Africa and parts of the Mediterranean, Middle East and India. Up to 40% of the population can be affected in some areas. Sickle-cell trait is thought to afford some protection against *Plasmodium falciparum* malaria and therefore HbS genes are positively selected in areas where malaria is endemic.

In HbS, a single base-pair substitution in codon 6 of the β-chain replaces glutamic acid with valine. Deoxygenated HbS is 50 times less soluble than deoxygenated HbA and it aggregates and polymerizes to form long intracellular fibres called tactoids. This causes elongation of the red cell into a rigid sickle shape. Reoxygenation can initially reverse the sickling process but, after repeated episodes, the red cells become irreversibly sickled.

HbS polymerizes best with other HbS molecules. The presence of other types of Hb (e.g. HbF or HbA) reduces sickling. Therefore sickle-cell anaemia is not apparent until approximately 6 months of age, when HbF levels fall. Individuals with sickle-cell trait are usually asymptomatic and those with sickle-cell haemoglobin C disease usually have clinically milder forms of the disease. There are four important syndromes associated with HbS:

1. Sickle-cell anaemia
2. Sickle-cell trait
3. Sickle-cell haemoglobin C disease
4. Sickle-cell β-thalassaemia.

Fig. 4.24 Features of sickle-cell anaemia

Feature	Notes
Chronic haemolytic anaemia	Non-deformable sickled cells are trapped in the splenic microcirculation, leading to premature cell death and the development of pigment gallstones
Infarctive or painful crises	Sickle cells lodge in small and medium sized blood vessels Precipitated by hypoxia, infection, acidosis, dehydration and cold Infected metacarpals and metatarsals cause dactylitis (hand–foot syndrome) in children Chronic tissue and organ damage ensues (bones, lungs, kidneys, liver and brain)
Haemolytic crises	Usually accompany infarctive crises
Aplastic crises	Due to parvovirus infection and to folate deficiency
Spleen	Enlarged in children due to trapped red cells but infarction leads to hyposplenism by ~6 years of age. Before the spleen is destroyed the patient is susceptible to potentially fatal splenic sequestration
Infections	Risk of overwhelming sepsis in early childhood—in asplenic state, more susceptible to infection with encapsulated organisms, e.g. *Streptococcus pneumoniae*—prone to *Salmonella* osteomyelitis
Other complications	Priapism, chronic leg ulcers, proliferative retinopathy
Laboratory findings	Hb 6–9 g/dL Reticulocytosis Sickle cells seen on blood film HbS detected on Hb electrophoresis; no HbA Red cells sickle upon mixing with sodium metabisulphite (sickling test) Sickle-cell haemoglobin is insoluble in a high molarity phosphate buffer

Hb, haemoglobin; HbA, adult haemoglobin; HbS, sickle haemoglobin.

Sickle-cell anaemia (homozygous for HbS, denoted $\beta^s\beta^s$) is the most serious of these. Features of sickle-cell anaemia are listed in Fig. 4.24. Management strategies include:

- Pneumococcal, meningococcal and Hib vaccines
- Penicillin prophylaxis
- Folic acid supplements
- Avoidance of factors precipitating infarctive crises
- Prompt treatment of infection
- Management of infarctive crises with fluids, analgesia (including opiates), warmth and antibiotics if necessary
- Blood transfusions and exchange transfusions when necessary
- Prevention of iron overload.

Sickle-cell trait (heterozygous, HbSA, $\beta^s\beta$) individuals are generally asymptomatic. Sickling occurs at very low partial pressures of oxygen that are rarely reached in vivo. Both HbA and HbS bands are detectable on electrophoresis but sickled cells are not usually seen. Haemoglobin solubility test is positive.

Sickle-cell haemoglobin C disease (HbS/HbC, $\beta^s\beta^c$) arises from carriage of two abnormal β genes. It is clinically similar to, but less severe than, sickle-cell anaemia. Patients are more susceptible to thrombosis and pulmonary embolism and are more likely to develop proliferative retinopathy.

Sickle-cell β-thalassaemia ($\beta^s\beta^0$ or $\beta^s\beta^+$) shares its clinical features with sickle-cell anaemia, but its severity is variable and depends on the amount of normal β-chain synthesis.

ANAEMIA DUE TO BLOOD LOSS

Acute blood loss

Causes of acute blood loss include trauma, surgery, peripartum haemorrhage, haematemesis and haemoptysis. Plasma volume is replaced within 1–3 days of the acute blood loss but it can take several weeks for the red cell mass, and therefore haemoglobin, to be replenished. Haematological findings in acute blood loss include:

- A normocytic, normochromic anaemia
- A reticulocytosis that peaks 1–2 weeks after the haemorrhage
- An increase in the number of platelets and neutrophils
- Neutrophil precursors in the peripheral blood.

Red-cell parameters might be normal before compensation for the loss of intravascular volume as both plasma and red cells have been lost in their normal proportions.

Chronic blood loss

The most common causes of chronic blood loss are gastrointestinal lesions and menorrhagia. The consequences are those of iron-deficiency anaemia (see p. 87).

Acquired defects of the red cell
Paroxysmal nocturnal haemoglobinuria (PNH)

This is a rare, acquired red-cell membrane defect. A mutation in the gene coding for phosphatidylinositol glycan protein A (PIG-A) leads to a lack of glycosyl phosphatidylinositol (GPI). GPI anchors certain proteins to the cell membrane. These proteins usually prevent lysis of blood cells by complement and their absence leads to chronic intravascular haemolysis. PNH is a stem cell disorder, so patients may have leucopenia and thrombocytopenia in addition to anaemia.

Antibody-mediated red-cell destruction
Autoimmune haemolytic anaemias

In the autoimmune haemolytic anaemias (AIHAs), red-cell autoantibodies cause haemolysis. A positive direct Coombs test can be demonstrated. There are three types of AIHA:

1. Warm AIHA (occurs at body temperature)
2. Cold AIHA (usually occurs below room temperature)
3. Paroxysmal cold haemoglobinuria.

Warm AIHA can be idiopathic or secondary to autoimmune disease (especially SLE), leukaemias (especially chronic lymphocytic leukaemia), lymphomas and drugs (e.g. methyldopa). The clinical features are as follows:

- Anaemia
- Jaundice
- Splenomegaly (almost always, although often very mild)
- Evans' syndrome, which is the combination of warm AIHA and idiopathic thrombocytopenic purpura (ITP) (very rare).

Identified causes should be eliminated. Patients generally respond well to steroids but other immunosuppressive therapies or splenectomy might also be required.

Cold AIHA can be idiopathic or secondary to lymphoma or infection (e.g. mycoplasma pneumonia, Epstein–Barr virus). The clinical features are as follows:

- Symptoms worse in cold weather
- Acrocyanosis (purplish discoloration of the skin) due to vascular sludging arising from red-cell agglutination
- Raynaud's phenomenon.

Treatment involves the elimination of any cause, the patient should be kept warm and immunosuppressive therapy should be considered.

Paroxysmal cold haemoglobinuria is a subset of cold AIHA in which haemolysis occurs at higher temperatures but antibody binding occurs at cold temperatures.

The laboratory features of warm and cold AIHAs are compared in Fig. 4.25.

Alloimmune haemolytic anaemias

Alloimmune haemolytic anaemias are caused by a reaction between antibodies and blood cells from different people. This occurs following:

- Transfusion of ABO-incompatible blood
- Transfer of maternal antibodies across the placenta in haemolytic disease of the newborn
- Allogeneic transplantation.

Drug-induced immune haemolytic anaemias

Certain drugs (e.g. penicillin, quinine and methyldopa) can precipitate haemolysis via a variety of immune mechanisms.

Fig. 4.25 Comparison of laboratory features of autoimmune haemolytic anaemias (AIHAs)

Feature	Warm AIHA	Cold AIHA	Paroxysmal cold haemoglobinuria
Antibody class	IgG	IgM	IgG (Donath–Landsteiner)
Antibody specificity	May be Rhesus	May be I or i antigens	Red cell P antigen
Antibody binding temperature	37°C	<32°C	<32°C
Red cell agglutination	✗	✓	✓
Complement fixation	✗	✓	✓
Mechanism of cell destruction	Mainly extravascular	Mainly intravascular	Mainly intravascular
Direct Coombs test	Positive for IgG and complement	Positive for complement	Positive for IgG and complement

Other causes of haemolysis

- Mechanical trauma:
  - classically with mechanical heart valves
  - microangiopathic haemolytic anaemia occurs when fibrin is deposited in small vessels. This is seen in haemolytic uraemic syndrome, thrombotic thrombocytopenic purpura, disseminated carcinoma, malignant hypertension and Gram-negative septicaemia. It is characterized by red cell fragments (schistocytes) in the blood film
  - march haemoglobinuria is caused by damage to red cells in the feet during long periods of walking or running. The blood film does not show fragments
- Chemicals and toxins, e.g. lead poisoning, some snake venoms
- Infection, e.g. malaria
- Hypersplenism.

Anaemia of chronic disease

This is a common type of anaemia seen in hospital (and therefore important to be able to understand and differentiate). It is associated with chronic infections, neoplasms and disorders of the immune system. The mechanism behind anaemia of chronic disease is complex but is thought to relate to activation of cellular immunity and the production of proinflammatory cytokines.

Activated macrophages are erythrophagocytic and secrete cytokines such as TNF which result in decreased erythropoiesis and red cell lifespan. The anaemia is usually normocytic and normochromic, although a microcytic hypochromic anaemia occurs in approximately one-third of cases.

Making the diagnosis of anaemia of chronic disease or iron-deficiency anaemia

If the MCV is exceptionally low (<70 fL), iron deficiency is the most likely cause.

The important concept to understand is that in anaemia of chronic disease there is no deficiency of iron, only a deficiency in the ability to utilize iron stores. Therefore serum iron is low in both conditions.

- Assessment of iron status in iron deficiency:
  - Serum iron: low
  - Ferritin: low
  - Serum transferrin: increased or normal
  - Serum transferrin receptors: increased
- Assessment of iron status in chronic disease:
  - Serum iron: low
  - Ferritin: increased or normal
  - Serum transferrin: decreased or normal
  - Serum transferrin receptors: decreased or normal.

The anaemia responds poorly to iron therapy and is correctable only by treatment of the underlying cause. EPO can help to increase erythrocyte production.

Fig. 4.26 Causes of aplastic anaemia	
Congenital	**Acquired**
Fanconi type—a rare autosomal recessive condition associated with other congenital anomalies and increased incidence of malignancy	• Idiopathic (50% of cases) • Drugs that cause marrow suppression (e.g. busulphan, chloramphenicol) • Ionizing radiation • Chemicals, e.g. benzene, insecticides • Infection, e.g. viral hepatitis • Paroxysmal nocturnal haemoglobinuria

Aplastic anaemia

Aplastic anaemia is characterized by pancytopenia and aplasia (hypocellularity) of the bone marrow. There is a reduction in the number of bone-marrow stem cells and those that remain are defective and cannot repopulate the marrow. Causes of aplastic anaemia are listed in Fig. 4.26. Treatment is supportive with removal of any causative factors. Specific treatment is with antilymphocyte globulin, ciclosporin, haemopoietic growth factors, androgens or stem cell transplantation.

Pure red-cell aplasia

This is a rare condition in which only the red-cell precursors in the bone marrow are defective. Parvovirus B19 causes transient red-cell aplasia.

Other forms of marrow failure

Space-occupying lesions can cause anaemia, e.g. metastatic carcinoma in the bone marrow, which destroys the bone marrow architecture.

Chronic renal failure is almost always associated with anaemia. A decreased renal mass results in reduced production of EPO.

POLYCYTHAEMIA (ERYTHROCYTOSIS)

Polycythaemia is an increase in haematocrit concentration above the normal upper limit for the patient's age and sex (0.51 in adult males and 0.48 in adult females).

Polycythaemia may be primary or secondary. Primary polycythaemia has no physiological benefit and arises from an abnormal clone of cells. Secondary polycythaemia occurs as a result of a physiological adaptation to hypoxia, with the erythrocytosis increasing the oxygen-carrying capacity of blood. A summary of the causes of polycythaemia is shown in Fig. 4.27.

Apparent polycythaemia can occur as a result of a reduction in the total plasma volume. Investigation to exclude this involves measuring total red cell volume (using ^{51}Cr) and total plasma volume (using ^{123}I-albumin).

Primary polycythaemia (polycythaemia rubra vera)

A proliferative abnormality of stem cells gives rise to increased numbers of red cells, often with an increase in the numbers of neutrophils and platelets. The red-cell precursors are inappropriately sensitive to insulin-like growth factor +/− interleukin-3 and therefore do not require EPO to avoid apoptosis. Haematological findings include:

• Raised packed cell volume, red-cell mass, haemoglobin and red-cell count
• Raised white-cell count (neutrophils and basophils)
• Raised neutrophil alkaline phosphatase
• Raised platelet count
• Hyperplasia of erythroid, granulocytic and megakaryocytic cells in bone marrow
• Decreased serum EPO
• Increased plasma urate
• Increased total blood volume and blood viscosity.

Fig. 4.27 Causes of polycythaemia

Absolute	Relative
Primary • Polycythaemia rubra vera (see text)	Fluid depletion • Dehydration (diarrhoea and vomiting) • Plasma loss, e.g. burns Cigarette smoking Stress (associated with smoking, alcohol, hypertension, obesity, diuretic therapy)
Secondary Appropriately increased erythropoietin: • High altitude • Chronic lung disease • Cyanotic heart diseases • Haemoglobin with abnormally high O_2 affinity Inappropriately increased erythropoietin: • Renal disease (carcinoma, cysts, transplants) • Hepatocellular carcinoma • Cerebellar haemangioblastoma • Massive uterine fibroids	

Polycythaemia rubra vera

Polycythaemia rubra vera presents insidiously after the age of 40, with symptoms attributable to hyperviscosity and vascular occlusion. These symptoms include:

- Headache
- Dizziness
- Stroke.

They are more likely to suffer from thrombosis than disorders of bleeding. Clinical signs include:

- Plethora
- Splenomegaly
- Hepatomegaly.

Treatment is by venesection reducing the packed cell volume to within normal limits. Other therapies include cytotoxic drugs (such as hydroxyurea) and irradiation of the bone marrow using ^{32}P. Some patients develop acute leukaemia or myelofibrosis. The main causes of death are thromboses and acute leukaemia. However, if the red-cell count is kept low, the prognosis is good.

Venesection as treatment for secondary polycythaemia should not aim to drastically reduce the packed cell volume as this negates the adaptive advantage of the compensatory erythropoiesis. Treatment should be to a level which reduces the symptoms caused by hyperviscosity (PCV approximately 0.55).

Recently a point mutation in the JAK2 gene has been shown by numerous studies to be associated with polycythaemia rubra vera. In some cases this finding may be of future use in making the diagnosis and as a target for treatments.

Objectives

You should be able to:

- Know the structure of the different classes of white blood cells, and how each is related to their specialized functions
- Discuss the mechanisms involved in leucocytosis
- Understand the processes involved in neoplastic proliferation of white blood cells
- Compare the differences between myeloid and lymphoid neoplasms
- Know the aetiology of Hodgkin's and non-Hodgkin's lymphoma
- Explain the different forms of myeloma
- Discuss the causes and features of leucopenia.

STRUCTURE AND FUNCTION OF THE WHITE BLOOD CELLS

See Chapter 1 for a discussion of the immunological functions of white blood cells.

Lymphocytes

Appearance and structure

Lymphocytes (Fig. 5.1) are the smallest white cells, 6–15 μm in diameter. In blood they are round but they can change shape outside the circulation. They have round, densely staining, acentric nuclei. The sparse cytoplasm contains a few lysosome-like granules. Once activated, the amount of cytoplasm increases. B cells and natural killer (NK) cells tend to be larger than T cells. The cells are differentiated by the presence of differing surface markers.

Location

Lymphocytes circulate between tissue, lymphatics and the blood. The lifespan of lymphocytes varies depending on their interaction with antigens. Memory cells can survive for decades.

Function

Lymphocytes have no functions in the blood, but are central to the adaptive immune response. They produce antibodies and kill foreign or virally altered cells.

Neutrophils

Appearance and structure

Neutrophils (Fig. 5.2), also known as polymorpho-nuclear leucocytes, measure 9–15 μm in diameter. They have distinctive nuclei containing 2–5 lobes connected by thin chromatin threads. In females, the nucleus has a 'drumstick' appendage that contains the inactivated X chromosome. Neutrophils have few mitochondria and large stores of glycogen. The cytoplasm contains an abundance of three types of granule:

1. Small, specific granules (0.1 μm in diameter) containing antimicrobial enzymes and other agents
2. Azurophilic granules (0.5 μm in diameter) similar to lysosomes
3. Tertiary granules containing gelatinase, cathepsins and glycoproteins.

Location

Neutrophils circulate in blood for up to 10 hours. In response to chemotactic agents they migrate into tissues, where they survive for 1–3 days.

97

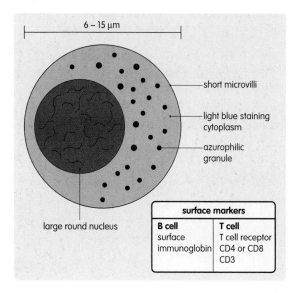

Fig. 5.1 Lymphocyte structure.

Fig. 5.3 Monocyte structure. MHC, major histocompatibility complex.

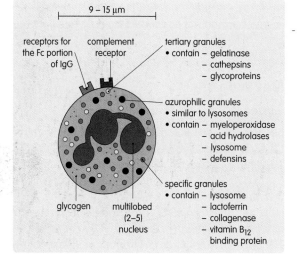

Fig. 5.2 Neutrophil structure.

Function

Neutrophils are the first cells to reach sites of inflammation and, once defunct, they are the major constituent of pus. They destroy microorganisms by phagocytosis and release of hydrolytic enzymes.

Monocytes

Appearance and structure

Monocytes (Fig. 5.3) tend to be the largest circulating blood cell, up to 25 μm in diameter. They have

a large, kidney-shaped nucleus. Nucleoli are often present, giving the nucleus a 'moth-eaten' appearance. The cytoplasm contains many lysosomes and vacuole-like spaces producing a 'ground-glass' appearance. Microtubules, microfilaments, pinocytotic vesicles and filo- or pseudopodia are present around the edge of the cell.

Location

Monocytes spend only a few days in the blood before migrating into the tissues, where they differentiate to become macrophages. Macrophages survive for several months to years in connective tissue.

Function

Monocytes form the reticuloendothelial system, which is primarily involved in phagocytosis. They destroy dead or defunct cells and ingest foreign material. Antigens are processed and can be presented to lymphocytes to initiate an adaptive immune response. Macrophages also have a proinflammatory function, releasing a variety of cytokines.

Eosinophils

Appearance and structure

Eosinophils (Fig. 5.4) are similar to neutrophils but larger: 12–17 μm in diameter. Their nucleus is

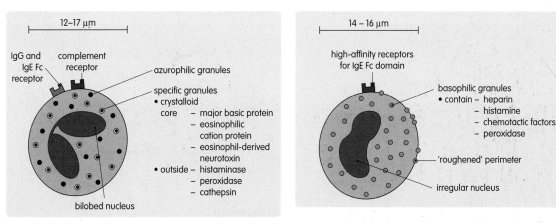

Fig. 5.4 Eosinophil structure.

Fig. 5.5 Basophil structure.

sausage-shaped and usually bilobed. They have a small, central Golgi apparatus and limited rough endoplasmic reticulum and mitochondria. Eosinophils contain large, ovoid, specific granules and azurophilic granules. The specific granules (1–1.5 μm long) have a crystalloid centre containing major basic protein, eosinophilic cationic protein and eosinophil-derived neurotoxin. The outside of the granule contains several enzymes, including histaminase, peroxidase and cathepsin.

Location

They are primarily found in the tissues, spending less than 1 hour in blood.

Function

Their primary function is to combat parasitic infection. Eosinophils also phagocytose antigen–antibody complexes.

Basophils
Appearance and structure

Basophils (Fig. 5.5) are 14–16 μm in diameter with a bilobed, 'S-shaped' nucleus. They are named after their highly basophilic cytoplasmic specific granules, but also contain azurophilic granules. Specific granules (0.5 μm in diameter) are large, membrane-bound, round or oval structures. They push into the plasma membrane causing a 'roughened perimeter'. The granules contain heparin, histamine, chemotactic factors and peroxidase.

Location

The lifespan is unknown; however, they survive for 1–2 years in mice.

Function

Basophils may be the precursors to mast cells, with which they share many similarities, but nowadays they are thought to be of two different lineages. Basophils are thought to mediate inflammatory responses.

DIFFERENTIATION OF WHITE CELLS

Granulocytes and monocytes are formed in the bone marrow from a common precursor cell (CFU-GM). Their differentiation pathways are shown in Fig. 5.6.

REACTIVE PROLIFERATION OF WHITE CELLS

Leucocytosis

Leucocytosis is an increase in the total white cell count (>11 × 10⁹/L). Fig. 5.7 outlines the numerical criteria for normal differential white-cell counts. One leucocyte type, most commonly neutrophils, tends to predominate, with small increases in other types. Diseases associated with increases in white-cell count are listed in Fig. 5.8.

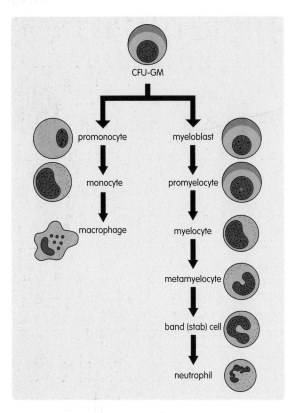

Fig. 5.6 Production of myeloid cells and monocytes. Eosinophils and basophils are formed by a process similar to the one shown for neutrophils. Neutrophils usually develop within bone marrow, but with increased demand, e.g. severe infection, band cells may be seen in blood. CFU-GM, granulocyte, monocyte colony-forming unit.

Fig. 5.7 Normal values for differential white-cell counts	
Cell type	**Normal levels**
Leucocytes	$4–11 \times 10^9$/L
Neutrophils	$2–7.5 \times 10^9$/L
Eosinophils	$0.04–0.44 \times 10^9$/L
Basophils	$0–0.1 \times 10^9$/L
Lymphocytes	$1.3–3.5 \times 10^9$/L
Monocytes	$0.2–0.8 \times 10^9$/L

Normal black and Middle Eastern people may have lower counts. Children younger than 12 years of age and pregnant women normally exhibit higher levels of white cells.

A general increase in white blood cells is called a leucocytosis and in lymphocytes is called a lymphocytosis; a specific increase in granulocyte counts is known as a granulocytosis. If neutrophils, eosinophils or basophils are selectively raised, then the terms neutrophilia, eosinophilia or basophilia are used, respectively.

Lymphadenopathy

The lymph nodes can become enlarged during any infective or inflammatory disease, but can be an important indicator of haematological disease. Acute presentation of rapidly expanding painful nodes is likely to be infectious. Slow growth of painless nodes is often haematological in origin. If lymphadenopathy is localized, the cause is more likely to be localized. Common causes of lymphadenopathy are shown in Fig. 5.9.

NEOPLASTIC PROLIFERATION OF WHITE CELLS

A neoplastic clone can arise at any stage in development, from the myeloid stem cell and in either one of the three lineages, with more mature cells involved less commonly.

Characteristically, the myeloproliferative disorders show an increased number of cells with normal morphology and function, whereas the myelodysplastic disorders are characterized by abnormal morphology (dysplasia) and function, and an increase in the number of blast cells.

Features common to leukaemias

Leukaemias are a group of disorders characterized by accumulation of abnormal blood cells in bone marrow. They are clonal disorders, i.e. they result from successive uncontrolled divisions of a single cell. The leukaemic 'blast' cells are non-functional and replace normal bone marrow, encroaching on normal haemopoietic cell development. This leads to:

- Anaemia
- Neutropenia
- Thrombocytopenia.

Fig. 5.8 Diseases associated with increased white-cell counts

Cell type	Associated diseases	Examples
Leucocytes	Pathological stress, leukaemia	
Neutrophils	Bacterial infections	Pyogenic bacteria
	Acute inflammation or tissue necrosis	Infarction, surgery, burns, myositis, vasculitis
	Neoplasms	Carcinoma, lymphoma, melanoma
	Myeloproliferative disorders	Chronic myeloid leukaemia, myelofibrosis
	Metabolic disorders	Eclampsia, gout, diabetic ketoacidosis
Eosinophils	Parasitic infestation	Malaria, hookworm, filariasis, schistosomiasis
	Allergic reaction	Asthma, hay fever
	Skin disease	Pemphigus, eczema, psoriasis, dermatitis herpetiformis, urticaria
	Neoplasms	Hodgkin's disease, metabolic carcinoma, chronic myeloid leukaemia
	Infections	Convalescent phase of any infection
Basophils	Myeloproliferative disorders	Chronic myeloid leukaemia, polycythaemia rubra vera
Lymphocytes	Acute infections	Infectious mononucleosis, pertussis, rubella, viral infection
	Chronic infections	TB, syphilis
	Neoplasms	Chronic lymphocytic leukaemia, lymphoma
Monocytes	Chronic infections and inflammatory diseases	TB, bacterial endocarditis, protozoa
	Neoplasms	Lymphomas, myelodysplastic syndromes

TB, tuberculosis.

Many symptoms of leukaemia are due to organ infiltration by leukaemic cells. Organs that are commonly involved include:
- Bones
- Lymph nodes
- Liver and spleen (might also be involved by extramedullary haemopoiesis)
- Skin
- Central nervous system.

Classification of leukaemia is based on:

- Cell lineage (lymphoid or myeloid)
- Developmental stage of leukaemic cells: acute leukaemia involves proliferation of immature cells (blasts) and, untreated, is usually rapidly fatal; chronic leukaemia involves more mature cells, and a more prolonged course is characteristic.

Acute leukaemias are myeloblastic (AML) or lymphoblastic (ALL). The French–American–British (FAB) classification (Fig. 5.10) further subdivides acute leukaemia into different groups based on their morphology and cytochemistry.

Myeloproliferative disorders

These disorders arise as a result of the neoplastic clonal proliferation of multipotent myeloid stem cells, which are capable of following one or more differentiation pathways (Fig. 5.11). Myeloproliferative disorders encompass:

- Primary polycythaemia (polycythaemia rubra vera)
- Myelofibrosis
- Primary thrombocythaemia.

Myelofibrosis

Chronic idiopathic myelofibrosis can be preceded by other myeloproliferative conditions; 25% of cases are preceded by polycythemia rubra vera. Bone marrow is replaced by fibrous tissue produced by fibroblasts in conjunction with proliferation of dysplastic megakaryocytes. Massive splenomegaly occurs due to extramedullary haemopoiesis. The disease affects individuals from middle-age onwards. Clinical features include constitutional symptoms of weight loss, night sweats and fever, or those relating to anaemia (fatigue, shortness of breath and palpitations) or splenomegaly (abdominal pain due to the mass effect). Laboratory features at presentation include anaemia, leucocytosis and thrombocytosis. The blood film is often diagnostic, revealing:

- Granulocyte precursor cells
- Nucleated red blood cell precursors
- Tear-drop poikilocytosis (tear-drop-shaped erythrocytes).

Supportive care (including transfusions of red cells) can be useful, and splenectomy or splenic irradiation is sometimes beneficial. Chemotherapy with hydroxyurea can slow or reverse fibrosis. Median survival is 3 years. Approximately 10% of cases transform into acute myeloblastic leukaemia (AML).

Primary thrombocythaemia

This is a disorder involving clonal proliferation of the megakaryocyte cell line, although it is really a stem cell disorder. A raised platelet count ($>600 \times 10^9$/L) is the dominant feature. It usually presents after the age of 50 but the incidence is increasing in younger women. About half of affected individuals are asymptomatic at diagnosis, thus it is often discovered as an incidental finding on routine blood test.

The disorder is characterized clinically by thrombosis or bleeding. Haemorrhage is more common with higher platelet counts, e.g. $>1000 \times 10^9$/L, and in those with acquired von Willebrand's disease (see p. 121). There are raised levels of abnormal megakaryocytes in the bone marrow. Splenic atrophy, as a result of microinfarcts, occurs in 50% of cases.

Fig. 5.9 Causes of lymphadenopathy

Cause	Example
Infective	*Streptococcus* spp. *Mycobacterium tuberculosis* Epstein–Barr virus HIV Toxoplasmosis Brucellosis Histoplasmosis Coccidioidomycosis
Neoplasia	Leukaemias Lymphomas Secondary, e.g. lung, breast
Connective tissue disease	Rheumatoid arthritis Systemic lupus erythematosus
Drugs	Phenytoin Para-aminosalicylic acid
Others	Sarcoidosis Amyloidosis

HIV, human immunodeficiency virus.

Fig. 5.10 The French–American–British (FAB) classification of acute leukaemias

Myeloblastic	Lymphoblastic
M0—undifferentiated myeloblastic leukaemia	L1—homogeneous population of small lymphoblasts
M1—acute myeloblastic leukaemia without maturation	L2—heterogeneous population of large lymphoblasts with one or more nucleoli
M2—acute myeloblastic leukaemia with maturation	L3—homogeneous population of large lymphoid cells with basophilic, vacuolated cytoplasm (now known as Burkitt's leukaemia/lymphoma)
M3—acute promyelocytic leukaemia	
M4—acute myelomonocytic leukaemia	
M5—acute monoblastic leukaemia	
M6—acute erythroleukaemia	
M7—acute megakaryoblastic leukaemia (rare)	

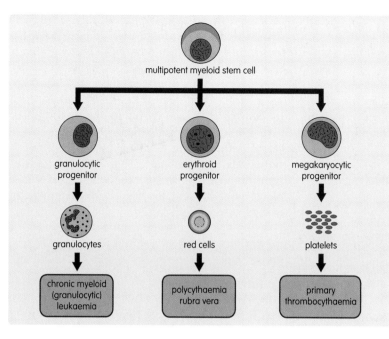

Fig. 5.11 Possible differentiation pathways of multipotent myeloid stem cells and associated myeloproliferative disorders.

Fig. 5.12 The French–American–British (FAB) classification of myelodysplastic syndromes

Type	Peripheral blood	Bone marrow
Refractory anaemia (RA)	Blasts <1%	Blasts <5%
Refractory anaemia with ringed sideroblasts (RARS)	Blasts <1%	Blasts <5%, ring sideroblasts >15% of total erythroblasts
RA with excess blasts (RAEB)	Blasts <5%	Blasts 5–20%
RAEB in transformation*	Blasts >5%	Blasts 20–30% or Auer rods present
Chronic myelomonocytic leukaemia (CMML)	Any above + >1.0 × 10⁹/L monocytes	Any above + promonocytes

Now often considered to be acute myeloid leukaemia.

Treatment involves the reduction of platelet levels by hydroxyurea or anagrelide. Aspirin is commonly used to reduce thrombotic risk.

Myelodysplastic syndromes

Myelodysplasias are acquired neoplastic disorders of bone marrow, with replacement of normal cells by a clone of abnormal (dysplastic) cells. These cells are unable to mature normally, usually affecting at least two cell lines (erythrocytes, granulocytes, monocytes or platelets) and as a result blast cells may accumulate. The dysmorphic cells are easily recognizable on microscopy with an increasing blast cell count indicating a poorer prognosis. Common features of myelodysplasias include:

- Occurs most commonly in the elderly and in males
- Slowly progressive disease, often with anaemia, easy bruising or bleeding and infections
- May follow chemo- and/or radiotherapy for another condition
- Normal or increased bone marrow cellularity
- Cytopenias
- Progression to AML.

The five myelodysplastic syndromes are classified in Fig. 5.12. Survival is best when blasts occupy less than 5% of the marrow.

Treatment until recently has been mainly supportive with blood and platelet transfusions. Younger patients with more advanced disease will be treated with intensive chemotherapy and possibly bone marrow transplantation. There is evidence that the use of biological therapy such as EPO and GM-CSF will improve survival in some patients. There may also be a role for thalidomide and its derivatives.

Acute myeloid leukaemia

Acute myeloid leukaemia (AML, sometimes called acute myeloblastic leukaemia) is the most common leukaemia in adults, although it can occur at any age. It is a clonal disorder of myeloid origin, producing primitive blast cells that invade bone marrow, suppressing all normal cell lines. These blast cells can be seen on peripheral blood films. The majority of cases have no known cause, although they can progress from both the myeloproliferative and myelodysplastic disorders. The incidence increases with age (median 60 years) with an average of 1 in 1000 per year. The 5-year survival rate is over 50% in children and about 30–50% in adults who are treated. Elderly patients have a poorer prognosis. AML is associated with:

- Radiation exposure
- Toxins: benzene, alkylating agents
- Hereditary abnormalities, e.g. Down syndrome
- Pre-existing haematological disease: chronic myeloid leukaemia (CML), myelodysplastic syndromes

but usually there is no obvious cause.

Patients are often acutely unwell at presentation and can present with:

- Anaemia, malaise, sweats, weight loss
- Infections (chest, mouth, skin)
- Bleeding
- Skin infiltration (gums M4/5)
- Leucostasis.

Leucostatic symptoms occur when white blood cells form thrombi in the heart, lungs and brain. Symptoms include reduced consciousness, retinal haemorrhages and pulmonary infiltrates.

Chromosome rearrangements have prognostic value with t(15;17), t(8;21) and inversion of 16 having better outcomes than monosomy 7.

AML is treated with combination chemotherapy, usually as part of national collaborative trials (alas, no longer by the Medical Research Council) and, in some cases, bone marrow transplantation. Survival is best in younger patients. The haematological consequences of AML are treated to improve symptoms and outcome. This includes transfusions of red cells/platelets, leukopheresis to reduce blood viscosity and the prevention/treatment of infection.

AML

Patients usually present with a short history of recurrent sore throats or easy bruising. A blood count reveals anaemia and thrombocytopenia. The WBC may be low or high but there will be blast cells in the bone marrow which may also be seen in the blood. These patients require immediate admission to hospital. If they are not treated with intensive chemotherapy they will rapidly die of sepsis or bleeding.

Chronic myeloid leukaemia

CML, also known as chronic granulocytic leukaemia, is a progressive accumulation of mature myeloid cells in blood and bone marrow. At presentation the white-cell count can be $300–500 \times 10^9$/L (normal levels are between 4 and 11×10^9/L), predominantly due to increases in myeloid cells. It accounts for 20% of all leukaemias. The average incidence is 1 in 100,000, peaking between 40 and 60 years of age. It is rare in children and there is a slight male preponderance. Clinically, it runs a predictable course, with three identifiable phases of the disease:

1. Chronic
2. Accelerated
3. Blast crisis (AML/ALL).

People normally present in the chronic phase following an incidental finding on a full blood count or with constitutional (malaise, weight loss, sweats) or leucostatic symptoms. Many patients will quickly transform to an accelerated or blast crisis stage, if untreated.

The Philadelphia chromosome is a pathognomonic translocation between chromosomes 9 and 22 associated with CML. This translocation, found in granulocytic, erythrocytic and megakaryocytic precursor cells, fuses parts of two genes (BCR-ABL) to create an abnormal tyrosine kinase, which is thought to be involved in disease progression. A tyrosine kinase inhibitor, imatinib (traded as Glivec), is now available and has greatly improved outcome for these patients. Bone marrow transplantation is potentially curative.

Median survival before the introduction of imatinib was 5½ years, but this should now improve. Good prognostic factors include:

- Youth
- Small spleen at presentation
- Low white-cell count at presentation.

Neoplasia of lymphoid origin
Acute lymphoblastic leukaemia

ALL accounts for 80% of all childhood leukaemias but is less common in adults. The peak incidence occurs between 2 and 10 years of age. Presentation outside of this range confers a poorer prognosis. ALL may be associated with:

- Radiation
- Chemicals
- Down syndrome

but usually there is no obvious cause.

In 80% of cases, the blast cells are of B cell origin. ALL is more responsive to combination chemotherapy than AML and long-term remission rates of over 70% are attained. Cure rates are highest in girls over 2 and under 10 years of age. The Philadelphia chromosome is seen in 10–20% of cases and is associated with a poor outcome.

Chronic lymphocytic leukaemia

CLL occurs most frequently in people over the age of 60 years (median age 65) and accounts for 20–50% of all leukaemias. It is twice as common in men as in women, with a total incidence of 3–4 per 10,000. CLL arises from a proliferation of neoplastic lymphoid cells (B cells), which infiltrate the marrow, lymph nodes, spleen and liver. It is a slowly progressing, low-grade disorder. Symptoms seen in other leukaemias are seen in 50% of CLL at diagnosis and associated autoimmune haemolytic anaemia is common.

On a blood film, leukaemic cells resemble mature lymphocytes, although typical 'smear cells' are also seen. Disease transformation into prolymphocytic leukaemia occurs rarely and usually after several years. Median survival is 5–8 years and treatment (chemotherapy or stem cell transplantation) is usually aimed at limiting rather than curing the disease. Many elderly patients will die of an unrelated condition because of the slowly progressive nature of the disease.

Hairy cell leukaemia

This condition causes pancytopenia due to monoclonal proliferation of a type of B cell with an irregular cytoplasmic outline. The number of 'hairy' cells in the peripheral blood is very variable; however, they are found in bone marrow. The peak incidence is 40–60 years of age, with males four times more likely than females to develop hairy cell leukaemia. Treatment with 2-chlorodeoxyadenosine or deoxycoformycin causes remission in >90% of cases and long-term survival is common.

Malignant lymphomas

Lymphomas are a group of neoplastic disorders characterized by the proliferation of a primitive cell to produce clonal expansion of lymphoid cells. They primarily involve the lymph nodes and extranodal lymphoid tissue, e.g. mucosal-associated lymphoid tissue (MALT) and spleen. Malignant lymphomas are divided into two categories:

1. Non-Hodgkin's lymphoma
2. Hodgkin's disease (Hodgkin's lymphoma).

Although it is easy to think of leukaemias as disease of the bone marrow and lymphomas as disease of the lymph nodes, remember that leukaemic cells are found in the blood and that lymphoma cells commonly spread to the bone marrow and blood.

Non-Hodgkin's lymphomas

Non-Hodgkin's lymphomas (NHL) are a group of malignant diseases involving lymphoid cells. NHL is classified into low-, intermediate- and high-grade disease in terms of clinical behaviour (Fig. 5.13).

Fig. 5.13 The Revised European American Lymphoma (REAL) classification of non-Hodgkin's lymphoma

Grade	B cell	T cell

Low	Small lymphocytic lymphoma
	Lymphoplasmacytic lymphoma/
	   Waldenström's macroglobulinaemia
	Marginal zone lymphomas
	Follicular lymphoma (grades I and II)
		Sezary's syndrome/mycosis fungoides
		Smouldering/chronic adult T cell
		   leukaemia/lymphoma

Intermediate	Mantle cell lymphoma Follicular lymphoma (grade III)	Peripheral T cell lymphoma Angioimmunoblastic lymphoma Angiocentric lymphoma Intestinal T cell lymphoma
High	Diffuse large B cell lymphoma Primary mediastinal B cell lymphoma Precursor B lymphoblastic Burkitt's lymphoma	Anaplastic large cell lymphoma Precursor T lymphoblastic Adult T cell leukaemia/lymphoma

Fig. 5.14 Features of non-Hodgkin's lymphoma

- Superficial, asymmetric, painless lymphadenopathy
- Fever, night sweats and weight loss
- Oropharyngeal involvement (5–10%)
- Cytopenias due to marrow failure or autoimmunity
- Abdominal disease (spleen, liver, MALT and retroperitoneal/mesenteric nodes)

MALT, mucosal-associated lymphoid tissue.

Incidence of NHL rises with age and is more common in men than in women. There are several aetiological factors associated with NHL, including:

- Infections, e.g. Epstein–Barr virus and human T cell lymphotrophic virus 1
- Immunodeficiency, e.g. immunosuppressive therapy, HIV
- Autoimmune disorders
- Irradiation and carcinogens
- Inherited disorders, e.g. ataxia telangiectasia, Fanconi's syndrome.

The incidence of NHL has increased since the 1970s, probably because of increases in the number of immunodeficient people. The features of NHL are outlined in Fig. 5.14.

Low-grade lymphomas

Follicle centre cell lymphomas are the most common type. Low-grade disease has a benign course and responds to treatment. It is difficult to eradicate and relapse is inevitable. Chemotherapy and monoclonal antibody therapy are often used. Survival is 7–10 years and patients tend to die from resistant disease, infection or transformation to a higher-grade lymphoma.

Intermediate-grade lymphomas

Mantle cell lymphomas are increasingly recognized as being intermediate grade. They do not respond well to treatment but progress rapidly (median survival 3 years).

High-grade lymphomas

Large cell lymphomas are the most common. They respond well to treatment (40–50% long-term survival) if localized but otherwise they are aggressive and rapidly progressive. The standard treatment regimen is known as CHOP (cyclophosphamide, adriamycin, vincristine and prednisolone).

Hodgkin's disease

Hodgkin's disease (HD) characteristically affects young people in the third and fourth decades of life and is slightly more common in men. There is a second peak of incidence in the elderly and it can occur in children. Diagnosis requires the presence of pathognomonic Reed–Sternberg (RS) cells or derivatives, typically mixed with a variable inflammatory infiltrate. Disease severity is directly proportional to the number of RS cells found in the lesions and indirectly linked to the number of lymphocytes in the lesions. The RS cells are neoplastic derivatives of B cells with a dysfunctional immunoglobulin gene. RS cells are bi- or multinucleated, with prominent eosinophilic nucleoli, giving an 'owl's-eye' appearance. The clinical features of HD are shown in Fig. 5.15.

Hodgkin's disease has been classified into four histological subtypes (Fig. 5.16). Although histological composition is an important prognostic factor, clinical staging (Ann Arbor staging) is the most accurate indicator of long-term prognosis in HD (Fig. 5.17). Treatment depends on stage. Stages IA and IIA receive radiotherapy, which cures 75–95%. Other stages receive combination chemotherapy over 6 months but only 50–65% are cured. Late complications of the disease include:

- Infertility
- Radiation pneumonitis
- Pulmonary fibrosis
- Secondary cancers, including AML.

Fig. 5.15 Clinical features of Hodgkin's disease

- Painless, non-tender lymphadenopathy: cervical then axillary nodes are most common, mediastinal in 10%
- Splenomegaly (rarely massive)
- Respiratory symptoms (mediastinal mass → superior vena cava obstruction)
- Pruritus
- Constitutional symptoms
  - weight loss
  - sweats
  - high swinging 'Pel-Ebstein' fever
  - alcohol-induced pain

Multiple myeloma

Multiple myeloma is a malignant proliferation of plasma cells in bone marrow, which produce a monoclonal paraprotein and/or light chain. The monoclonal immunoglobulin is found in serum, whereas the light chain or Bence Jones protein is found in urine. These monoclonal proteins form a discrete band on the electrophoretic strip (Fig. 5.18).

The incidence of multiple myeloma is 4–6/100,000 a year. It is a disease of late middle age and the elderly. Survival with adequate treatment (combination chemotherapy, thalidomide, localized radiotherapy) is 3–5 years on average but this is highly variable and is improving with new treatment regimes. The aetiology is unknown, apart from an increased incidence related to exposure to ionizing radiation. Tumour necrosis factor and interleukin-6 have been implicated in initiation of disease.

Diagnosis requires two out of three of the following:

- Monoclonal paraprotein in serum or urine
- >10–15% of bone marrow to be plasma cells
- Osteolytic bone lesions on skeletal survey.

Clinical features

- Bone destruction such as diffuse osteoporosis and pathological fractures are a common feature. They are thought to arise as a result of bone resorption induced by the production of osteoclast-activating factor (OAF) by the myeloma cells (see Fig. 5.19 for the radiographic appearance of multiple myeloma)

Fig. 5.16 Rye classification of Hodgkin's disease (HD)

Lymphocyte predominant	10% of cases of HD. The infiltrate consists of large numbers of lymphocytes and histiocytes, interspersed with a few RS cells. This subtype has a good prognosis
Nodular sclerosing	50% of cases of HD and, unlike other forms of HD, is more common in women. Broad bands of collagen fibres divide the lymph node into nodules containing a mixture of lymphocytes, eosinophils, plasma cells, macrophages and lacunar cells
Mixed cellularity	30% of cases of HD. It is characterized by an infiltrate of histiocytes, plasma cells and eosinophils. Fewer lymphocytes and more RS cells are present than in the lymphocyte-predominant form of the disease
Lymphocyte depletion	10% of cases of HD. RS cells or their variants are present in large numbers in conjunction with relatively few lymphocytes. Lymphocyte depletion has the poorest prognosis of all forms of HD

RS, Reed–Sternberg.

Fig. 5.17 Ann Arbor staging of malignant lymphomas

Stage	Sites of involvement
I	Disease limited to single region of nodes or one extranodal site
II	Disease at two sites on the same side of the diaphragm
III	Disease at several sites on both sides of the diaphragm (includes spleen)
IV	Spread of disease to extralymphatic structures, e.g. bone marrow, gut, lung, liver

A: no symptoms
B: weight loss, sweats, fever

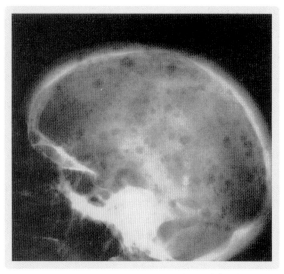

Fig. 5.19 A radiograph of the skull of a patient with multiple myeloma showing many osteolytic bone lesions (courtesy Dr M Makris).

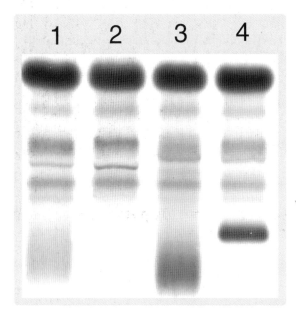

Fig. 5.18 Serum electrophoresis. Lane 1, normal sample; lane 2, patient with antibody deficiency; lane 3, patient with infection and polyclonal raised immunoglobulins; lane 4, patient with myeloma and monoclonal immunoglobulin.

- Neurological symptoms due to the compression of the spinal cord or roots by collapsed vertebrae
- Normochromic normocytic anaemia results from marrow infiltration
- Repeated infections can occur due to hypogammaglobulinaemia and neutropenia
- Hypercalcaemia occurs in 10% of cases. This is due to increased reabsorption of bone and is indicative of advanced disease

- Chronic renal failure occurs in 20–30% of patients. Factors that can contribute to renal failure in multiple myeloma are:
  - increased blood viscosity
  - hypercalcaemia
  - renal tubular obstruction by proteinaceous casts
  - toxic effect of Bence Jones protein on proximal renal tubules
  - infection
  - dehydration
  - non-steroidal anti-inflammatory drugs
  - light-chain deposition in glomeruli
- Amyloidosis (see below) can lead to nephrotic syndrome
- An abnormal bleeding tendency occurs owing to the adverse effect of paraprotein on platelets and coagulation factors.

Solitary myeloma (plasmacytoma)

A plasmacytoma is a solitary tumour found either in the bone or soft tissues, especially the upper respiratory tract. Osseous plasmacytomas usually progress to multiple myeloma. Extraosseous plasmacytomas do not disseminate and, after excision and radiotherapy, prognosis is excellent.

Waldenström's macroglobulinaemia

Waldenström's macroglobulinaemia is a neoplastic monoclonal proliferation of cells derived from the B-cell lineage. A monoclonal IgM paraprotein (macroglobulin) is produced, increasing blood viscosity markedly. Tumour cells are found in blood, bone marrow, lymph nodes and spleen. The incidence is 3–6/100,000 a year and is higher in males than in females. Most patients present between the fifth and seventh decade. Survival averages 2–5 years. Bone pain and osteolytic lesions are rare but hyperviscosity syndrome is common. Macroglobulin interferes with platelet function and coagulation factors, resulting in a tendency to bleed.

Heavy chain disease

Heavy chain disease is a rare condition where tumour cells secrete incomplete immunoglobulin heavy chain. This is most commonly α heavy chain disease (seen in Mediterranean countries). Heavy chain disease can progress to lymphoma.

Monoclonal gammopathy of undetermined significance

Around 3% of people aged over 65 years have low levels of paraprotein without any symptoms of disease. This condition is termed monoclonal gammopathy of uncertain significance (MGUS). There are <10% plasma cells in the marrow, no bone lesions, no anaemia and no renal failure; 10% will progress to myeloma within 10 years.

Amyloidosis

Amyloid is a heterogeneous group of proteins that have a fibrillar ultrastructure resulting in the formation of β-pleated sheets. Examples of amyloid proteins include:

- AA: serum amyloid A (SAA), an acute phase protein
- AL: immunoglobulin light chain or fragments.

In amyloidosis, amyloid is deposited in tissues. This can be localized or systemic, with renal impairment being a problem. Amyloidosis can occur in the following conditions:

- Chronic inflammatory disease (in which SAA is initially produced as an acute phase response protein)

- Primary disease
- Plasma cell disorders (multiple myeloma, Waldenström's macroglobulinaemia)
- Long-term haemodialysis
- Hereditary (very rare)
- Medullary carcinoma of the thyroid
- Ageing (cardiac or Alzheimer's disease).

LEUCOPENIA

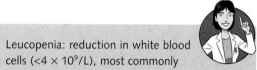

- Leucopenia: reduction in white blood cells ($<4 \times 10^9$/L), most commonly neutrophils
- Neutropenia (granulocytopenia): reduction in neutrophils ($<1.8 \times 10^9$/L)
- Agranulocytosis: severe, acute reduction in neutrophils ($<0.5 \times 10^9$/L in peripheral blood). Is associated with risk of infection and can be fatal
- Lymphopenia: reduction in lymphocyte count ($<1.5 \times 10^9$/L).

Causes of neutropenia and agranulocytosis

- Inadequate granulopoiesis
- Accelerated removal of granulocytes
- Drug-induced neutropenia.

Inadequate granulopoiesis

Reduced or ineffective production of neutrophils in the bone marrow results in neutropenia. This can be generalized bone marrow failure such as:

- Aplastic anaemia (see p. 95): a group of disorders characterized by anaemia, thrombocytopenia and neutropenia
- Invasion of the bone marrow in leukaemias and lymphomas. Neutropenia is accompanied by anaemia and thrombocytopenia
- Megaloblastic anaemia due to vitamin B_{12} or folate deficiency (see p. 87): this leads to impaired DNA synthesis, resulting in abnormal granulocyte precursors that are more susceptible to destruction

Fig. 5.20 Drugs that can cause neutropenia

- Analgesic and anti-inflammatory agents (aminopyrine, phenylbutazone)
- Hypnotics and sedatives (clozapine, mianserin, imipramine)
- Antimalarials (chloroquine)
- Diuretics and antihypertensives (furosemide)
- Anticonvulsants (phenytoin, carbamazepine)
- Antithyroid drugs (carbimazole)
- Antibiotics (chloramphenicol, co-trimoxazole, imipenem)
- Hypoglycaemic agents (tolbutamide)
- Antirheumatoid drugs (gold, sulfasalazine)

- Chemotherapy
- Myelodysplasia.

Or a specific failure of neutrophil production:

- Congenital (Kostmann's syndrome)
- Exposure to certain drugs (Fig. 5.20)
- Cyclical.

Accelerated removal of granulocytes

- Immune-mediated destruction:
  - idiopathic
  - secondary to other autoimmune diseases, e.g. Felty's syndrome (rheumatoid arthritis associated with leucopenia and splenomegaly)
  - due to drug therapy, e.g. chlorpromazine
  - hypersensitivity and anaphylaxis
- Hypersplenism causing splenic sequestration of neutrophils

- Severe infection (e.g. typhoid, miliary tuberculosis) resulting in increased peripheral utilization.

Drug-induced neutropenia

Drug-induced neutropenia is increasing in frequency. Two mechanisms operate:

1. Direct toxicity: interference with protein synthesis or cell replication of pluripotent stem cells causes a dose-dependent, generalized bone marrow depression
2. Immune-mediated destruction of neutrophils (see drug-induced immune destruction of red cells, p. 93): this is not related to drug dose and usually occurs early in the course of the therapy.

Causes of lymphopenia

The causes of lymphopenia are:

- Corticosteroid and other immunosuppressive therapy
- Trauma or surgery
- Cushing's syndrome
- Systemic lupus erythematosus (SLE)
- Hodgkin's lymphoma
- AIDS.

Mild lymphopenia has little in the way of clinical consequences and it is only in situations of prolonged severe lymphopenia, such as that seen in HIV-positive patients, where significantly clinical sequelae are evident.

You should be able to:

- Understand the structure and function of platelets, and how they are formed
- Explain different disorders affecting platelets
- Outline the different pathways and substances involved in the coagulation cascade
- Know how anticoagulants work, including the mechanisms of warfarin and heparin
- Understand the function and disorders of clotting factors
- Discuss different forms of thrombosis and how they arise.

When a defect such as trauma, inflammation or neoplasia occurs in a vascular wall, bleeding into the vessel wall and surrounding tissues takes place immediately. In normal people, a series of predetermined molecular events (haemostatic response) is initiated.

Haemostatic response: the arrest of bleeding, involving the physiological processes of platelet adhesion, blood coagulation and the contraction of damaged blood vessels.

Three local mechanisms are employed to try to avoid blood loss:

1. Local neurohumoral factors, such as endothelin released by cells adjacent to the injury, induce transient vasoconstriction
2. Primary haemostasis utilizes circulating platelets to form an adhesive plug to slow bleeding
3. Secondary haemostasis (the coagulation cascade) involves circulating plasma proteins. They produce a fibrin network that stabilizes the platelets and traps both red and white blood cells. This stable plug remains until cellular processes repair the damage.

PLATELETS AND BLOOD COAGULATION

Platelets are disc-shaped, non-nucleated, granule-containing cell fragments with a mean diameter of 2–3 µm (Fig. 6.1). They are formed in the bone marrow from megakaryocyte cytoplasm. The normal lifespan of platelets is 7–10 days and at any time up to a third are sequestered in the spleen.

Platelet structure and production

The normal discoid circulating shape is maintained by a band of 10–15 parallel microtubules located around the circumference. Platelets have two tubular systems: the dense tubular system and the surface-opening canalicular system. Platelets contain two types of granule, α and δ, which contain molecules involved in platelet aggregation.

Haemopoietic stem cells differentiate to form megakaryoblasts (Fig. 6.2). Megakaryoblasts mature by endomitosis, expanding cytoplasmic volume and increasing the number of nuclear lobes without dividing. This forms a polyploid megakaryocyte, which can produce 2000–7000 platelets. Cytoplasmic processes protrude into sinusoids where they fragment into proplatelets, which then disperse as individual platelets. Platelet production is controlled by:

- Negative feedback: number of circulating platelets
- Thrombopoietin release: increases platelet numbers
- Interleukin-3 (IL-3) and granulocyte–macrophage colony-stimulating factor (GM-CSF)—these stimulate CFU-megakaryocytes (CFU-MK).

Platelet functions

The main functions of platelets are adhesion, release reaction, aggregation, procoagulation and tissue repair.

111

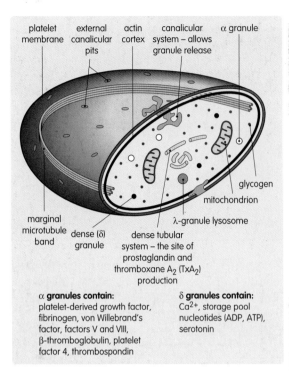

Fig. 6.1 Platelet structure. ADP, adenosine diphosphate; ATP, adenosine triphosphate, Ca²⁺, calcium ions.

α granules contain: platelet-derived growth factor, fibrinogen, von Willebrand's factor, factors V and VIII, β-thromboglobulin, platelet factor 4, thrombospondin

δ granules contain: Ca²⁺, storage pool nucleotides (ADP, ATP), serotonin

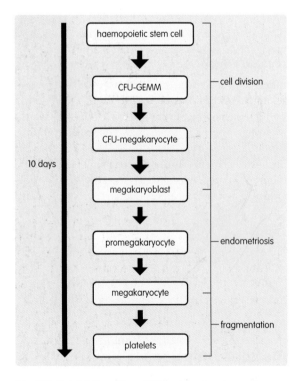

Fig. 6.2 Platelet formation. CFU, colony-forming unit; CFU-GEMM, granulocyte, erythrocyte, monocyte, megakaryocyte colony-forming unit.

Adhesion

Normally, endothelial cells have antiplatelet, anticoagulant and fibrinolytic activity. However, as blood oozes through defective vessel walls, platelets become exposed to the extracellular matrix of subendothelial vessel structures. This allows glycoprotein binding and platelet activation. Platelet plasma membrane glycoproteins are essential in mediating platelet interactions with other platelets or subendothelial connective tissue (Fig. 6.3). Examples of glycoprotein (GP) binding are as follows:

- GPIa: binds collagen
- GPIb: exists in complexes with GPV and GPIX and binds von Willebrand's factor (vWF). vWF, synthesized by endothelial cells and megakaryocytes, also binds exposed microfibrils
- GPIIb/IIIa: binds either vWF or fibrinogen.

Release reaction

Within 1–2 seconds of adhesion, a monolayer of platelets forms. Platelets change from discs to spheres with numerous cytoplasmic projections, promoting platelet–platelet interactions. Granule contents are released through the canalicular system.

Platelet aggregation

Granule contents promote further platelet adhesion and aggregation.

1. ADP, from δ granules, alters the surface configuration of locally circulating platelets, which promotes aggregation
2. Subendothelial collagen and thrombin promote ADP release and thromboxane A₂ (TxA₂) production, which potentiate platelet adhesion and aggregation
3. GPIIb/IIIa, exposed on aggregated platelets, binds plasma fibrinogen and promotes aggregation with platelets bound to the subendothelium, vWF and collagen
4. These interactions set up a cycle of further platelet aggregation and release of ADP and TxA₂, resulting in the formation of a platelet plug
5. Thrombin converts fibrinogen to fibrin, strengthening the platelet plug.

Prostacyclin (PGI₂), from endothelial cells, inhibits platelet aggregation and interactions with normal

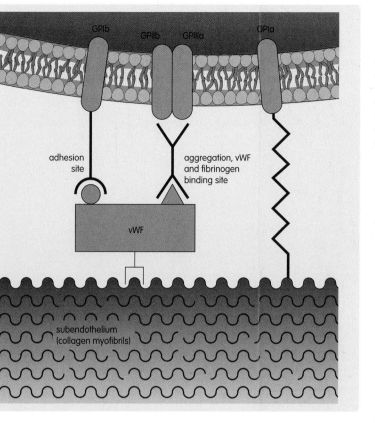

Fig. 6.3 Platelet adhesion reactions. von Willebrand's factor (vWF) binds to damaged vessel walls via subendothelial microfibrils. vWF interacts with platelets via GPIb (calcium required). This leads to exposure of GPIIIb/IIa receptor, which also binds vWF. Platelets bind directly to subendothelial collagen (types I, II and III) via GPIa.

endothelium (Fig. 6.4). Aggregation is made irreversible by:

- High levels of ADP
- Platelet-release products
- Platelet contractile proteins.

Procoagulant function

Platelet aggregation rearranges membrane phospholipid, forming an ideal site for coagulation reactions to take place (see the coagulation pathway, p. 116).

Tissue repair

Platelets stimulate wound healing through platelet-derived growth factor (PDGF), which is mitogenic for vascular smooth muscle cells and fibroblasts.

PLATELET DISORDERS

The normal concentration of platelets in blood is $150–400 \times 10^9$/L. A reduced platelet count (throm-

bocytopenia) or defects of platelet function can cause a disorder of bleeding (Fig. 6.5).

Reduced platelet count (thrombocytopenia)

Decreased platelet production

This is the most common cause of thrombocytopenia. The causes are listed in Fig. 6.6.

Generalized disease of the bone marrow

Decreased megakaryocyte production, and therefore platelet production, can be part of a wider clinical picture. Aplastic anaemia is associated with generalized bone marrow failure. Bone marrow infiltration, e.g. due to metastatic carcinoma, also reduces the number of marrow megakaryocytes.

Specific impairment of platelet production

Drugs (thiazide diuretics, ethanol and cytotoxics) can cause thrombocytopenia by several mechanisms:

- Depressing the whole bone marrow
- Specifically impairing megakaryocyte development or proliferation

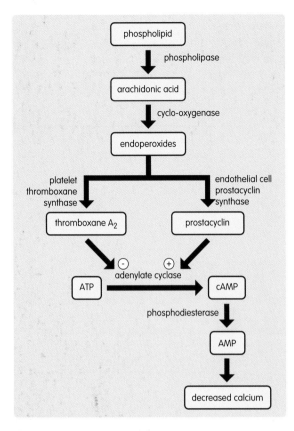

Fig. 6.4 The actions of prostacyclin and thromboxane A$_2$. AMP, adenosine monophosphate; ATP, adenosine triphosphate; cAMP, cyclic adenosine monophosphate.

Fig. 6.6 Causes of reduced platelet production	
Mechanism	Cause
Bone marrow failure	Aplastic anaemia
Bone marrow infiltration	• Metastatic carcinoma • Leukaemia • Lymphoma • Multiple myeloma • Myelofibrosis
Impaired platelet production	• Thiazides • Co-trimoxazole • Phenylbutazone • Alcohol • Chemo- or radiotherapy • Viruses, e.g. measles, HIV
Ineffective megakaryopoiesis	• Megaloblastic anaemia • Myelodysplasia

HIV, human immunodeficiency virus.

presses megakaryocytes, causing thrombocytopenia in 50% of patients.

Ineffective megakaryopoiesis

Impaired DNA synthesis in megaloblastic anaemia due to vitamin B$_{12}$ or folate deficiency results in ineffective thrombopoiesis.

Decreased platelet survival

The causes of decreased platelet survival are listed in Fig. 6.7.

Immune destruction

Acute idiopathic thrombocytopenic purpura (ITP) is a self-limiting, postviral illness most common in under 10 year olds. The platelet count is usually less than 20×10^9/L. It is hypothesized that the immune response following an infection results in circulation of antibody–viral antigen complexes. The complexes bind to platelets, which are subsequently removed by the reticuloendothelial system. Over 80% of patients recover without treatment, but in 5–10% of cases a chronic form of the disease develops (chronic ITP).

ITP in adults occurs predominantly between the ages of 15 and 50 years. The incidence is greater in women than in men. Patients present with petechiae, ecchymoses, epistaxis and menorrhagia. The platelet count can be very low ($20–80 \times 10^9$/L). The onset is usually insidious, with no history of a recent viral infection. Platelets are bound by IgG

Fig. 6.5 Platelet count and bleeding tendency	
Platelet count ($\times 10^9$/L)	Bleeding tendency
100–150	Normal haemostasis (if normal function)
20–100	Bleeding time increases: platelet transfusions might be required to cover trauma or surgery
<20	Risk of spontaneous bleeding from skin and mucous membranes and into the brain, pulmonary cavity and retina: prophylactic platelet transfusions to be considered

• Drug-dependent antiplatelet antibody formation (rare).

Viruses can impair platelet production by invading the megakaryocyte, e.g. measles. HIV precipitates the development of antiplatelet antibodies and sup-

Fig. 6.7 Causes of decreased platelet survival

Mechanism	Cause
Immune-mediated destruction	• Idiopathic thrombocytopenic purpura • Neonatal alloimmune thrombocytopenia • Post-transfusion purpura • Drugs, e.g. quinine, rifampicin • Associated with systemic lupus erythematosus, chronic lymphocytic leukaemia or lymphoma
Infections	• Bacterial sepsis, measles, rubella, influenza • HIV • Malaria
Non-immune	• Thrombotic thrombocytopenic purpura • Dilutional loss • Splenomegaly • Disseminated intravascular coagulation

HIV, human immunodeficiency virus.

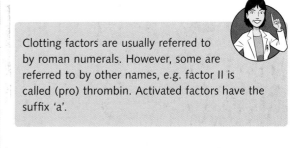

Clotting factors are usually referred to by roman numerals. However, some are referred to by other names, e.g. factor II is called (pro) thrombin. Activated factors have the suffix 'a'.

autoantibodies to platelet glycoproteins. The IgG–platelet complexes are removed by splenic macrophages, causing thrombocytopenia. If complement also binds, destruction mainly occurs in the liver. Adult onset ITP can be seen in conjunction with disorders causing aberrant immune responses, such as SLE. Adult onset ITP resolves spontaneously less commonly than in children and is characteristically relapsing and remitting.

Neonatal alloimmune thrombocytopenia is associated with the transfer of antiplatelet antibodies across the placenta, from the mother to the fetus. The commonest cause is when the platelets of the fetus express PLA1 and the mother's platelets do not.

Post-transfusion purpura occurs if donor platelets, but not recipient platelets, express the antigen PLA1. Antibodies and thrombocytopenia develop 5–10 days after a transfusion, although the reason for the destruction of the recipient's platelets is unclear.

Drug-induced immune thrombocytopenia occurs via a variety of mechanisms. The platelet count is often less than $10 \times 10^9/L$ and patients present with acute purpura. Drugs known to induce immune thrombocytopenia, e.g. quinine, should be stopped if the patient becomes thrombocytopenic.

Non-immune destruction

Thrombotic thrombocytopenic purpura (TTP) is a rare but serious disorder that most commonly, affects young adults. It is marked by fever, haemolysis, transient neurological defects and renal failure. Microthrombi (platelets and fibrin) are deposited in arterioles and capillaries, causing thrombocytopenia and microangiopathic haemolytic anaemia (erythrocytes fragment as they circulate through the partially occluded vessels). The aetiology of TTP is related to the pathology affecting the von Willebrand factor cleaving protease ADAMTS-13. Often TTP is due to a congenital defect in the ADAMTS-13 molecule.

Haemolytic–uraemic syndrome (HUS) is a disorder similar to TTP that affects infants and young children. However, in HUS the platelet–fibrin microthrombi are limited to the kidneys. In many patients, the disease follows recent infections with *Escherichia coli* or other enteric pathogens.

Disseminated intravascular coagulation

See page 123.

Splenic sequestration

In a normal individual, about 30% of total body platelets are in the spleen at any one time. These are freely exchangeable with those in the circulation. An increase in splenic size (splenomegaly) causes the splenic platelet pool to increase to the point that it may account for up to 90% of total body platelets, resulting in peripheral thrombocytopenia.

Dilutional thrombocytopenia

Whole blood that has been stored for more than 24 hours contains very few viable platelets, owing to their short half-life. Massive transfusion (>10 units/24 hours) of this platelet-poor blood can result in dilutional thrombocytopenia and also deficiency of most clotting factors.

Fig. 6.8 Causes of defective platelet function

	Type	Causes
Congenital	Defective adhesion	Bernard–Soulier syndrome
	Defective aggregation	Glanzmann's thrombasthenia
	Defective secretion	Storage pool diseases
Acquired		Aspirin therapy Uraemia

Fig. 6.9 The clotting cascade. The roman numerals indicate the different clotting factors.

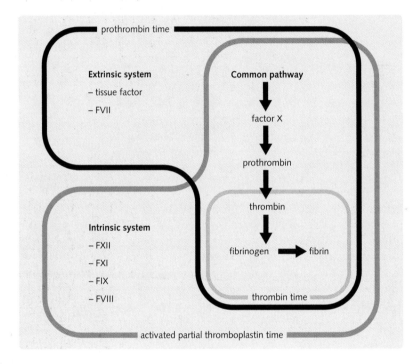

Defects of platelet function

These can be congenital or acquired (Fig. 6.8).

THE COAGULATION CASCADE

The coagulation pathways

The coagulation pathway (secondary haemostasis) involves a cascade of protein activation leading to the conversion of fibrinogen to fibrin. The proteins involved are known as clotting or coagulation factors. Coagulation can be initiated from within the circulation (intrinsic) or outside the circulation (extrinsic). An overview of the coagulation pathway is shown in Fig. 6.9.

The coagulation cascade is an amplification system that generates thrombin. Thrombin converts fibrinogen into fibrin and therefore stabilizes the clot. The factors required for coagulation are normally found in the circulation as proenzymes or cofactors (Fig. 6.10). The enzymes, except factor (F) XIII, are serine proteases that hydrolyse peptide bonds, amplifying the response. The coagulation factors adhere to activated platelets, e.g. the primary platelet plug. The platelet surface functions as a catalytic membrane for complexes of coagulation factors and is essential for the speed and magnitude of the secondary coagulation response.

Fig. 6.10 The coagulation factors

Factor number	Name	Active form
I	Fibrinogen	Fibrin
II	Prothrombin	Serine protease
V	Labile factor	Cofactor
VII	Proconvertin	Serine protease
VIII	Antihaemophilic factor	Cofactor
IX	Christmas factor	Serine protease
X	Stuart–Prower factor	Serine protease
XI	Plasma thromboplastin antecedent	Serine protease
XII	Hageman factor	Serine protease
XIII	Fibrin stabilizing factor	Transglutaminase
Prekallikrein		Serine protease
High-molecular-weight kininogen (HMWK)		Cofactor

The extrinsic pathway

The secondary haemostatic response is initiated by tissue factor (TF), a glycoprotein expressed on the surface of cells, such as monocytes, after tissue injury or inflammation. The activation of the coagulation cascade by TF is known as the 'extrinsic' pathway because the circulation is not normally exposed to TF. TF forms a complex with FVIIa, to produce a complex that activates both FX and FIX. FXa is important early in the coagulation cascade. In the presence of the cofactor FVa, FXa activates prothrombin, converting it to thrombin. Thrombin has many functions, including:

- Conversion of fibrinogen to fibrin
- Activation of factors V, VIII, XI and XIII
- Cleaving FVIII from vWF
- Further platelet activation
- Binding to thrombomodulin which then activates protein C.

A plasma protein called tissue factor pathway inhibitor (TFPI) binds to and prevents the TF–FVIIa complex activating FX but not FIX. The activation of cofactor VIII by thrombin allows FIXa to convert FX molecules to FXa. Cofactor V, also activated by thrombin, then aids the formation of more thrombin by FXa. The FIXa/FVIIIa complex is responsible for the continuous FXa formation and subsequent fibrin formation, which is essential for the formation of a durable secondary haemostatic plug.

Prothrombin time (PT) is used to test the extrinsic pathway. Tissue thromboplastin and calcium are added to citrated plasma. A normal clotting time is 10–14 seconds, but the value is normally given as an international normalized ratio (INR) which corrects for the variability between laboratories. Activated partial thromboplastin time (APPT) measures the intrinsic pathway. Phospholipid, a surface activator, and calcium are added to citrated plasma. A normal value is 30–40 seconds.

The intrinsic pathway

The 'intrinsic' pathway begins entirely within the circulation. Reactions between FXII, kallikrein and high-molecular-weight kininogen (HMWK) activate FXI. However, individuals with deficiencies of FXII, kallikrein and HMWK do not exhibit abnormal bleeding. Therefore the physiological role of the intrinsic pathway is uncertain and FXII is not generally considered to be a clotting factor. Intrinsic activation of FXI in major trauma and surgery may be important.

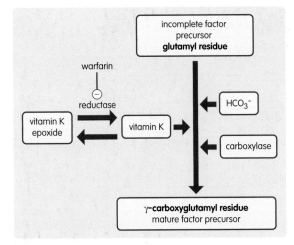

Fig. 6.11 Post-translational modification of the vitamin-K-dependent factors (factors II, VII, IX, X, proteins C and S). HCO_3^-, bicarbonate ions.

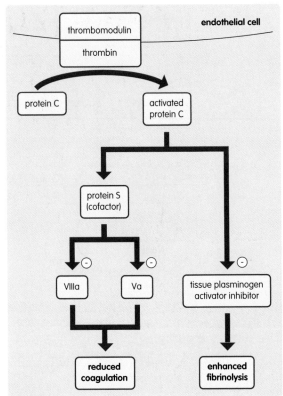

Fig. 6.12 Actions of proteins C and S to limit thrombus formation.

Fibrin

The final step of the secondary coagulation process is the degradation of the plasma protein fibrinogen into small fibrin monomers. These fibrin monomers polymerize spontaneously, by hydrogen bonds, to form long fibres and subsequent complex networks around the primary platelet plug. FXIIIa further stabilizes the clot by forming covalent cross-links between the fibrin polymers.

Role of vitamin K

Factors II, VII, IX and X undergo post-translational γ-carboxylation of glutamic acid residues. The modification of these factors allows them to bind calcium ions and platelet phospholipid membranes. The process, outlined in Fig. 6.11, requires vitamin K as a cofactor. Vitamin K is fat soluble and deficiency is often a result of malabsorption.

Role of calcium

Adequate levels of calcium are needed to allow clotting, by activating the vitamin-K-dependent factors. Reducing calcium within the test tube can prevent coagulation of blood samples. This is done by:

- Citrate → deionizes calcium
- Ethylenediaminetetraacetic acid (EDTA) → precipitates calcium.

Regulatory pathways

A complex regulatory system prevents extension of coagulation outside the site of injury.

Proteins C and S

Protein C is a serine protease that destroys the activated cofactors Va and VIIIa. It also enhances fibrinolysis by inhibiting tissue plasminogen activator inhibitor (PAI). Protein C is activated when thrombin binds to thrombomodulin on endothelial cells. Protein S is a cofactor for protein C (Fig. 6.12). Both proteins C and S are dependent on vitamin K (see Fig. 6.11).

Antithrombin III

Antithrombin III (ATIII) is a potent inhibitor of thrombin, FIXa, FXa and FXIIa. ATIII binds to the serine residue in the active site of these factors. The inhibitory effect of ATIII is potentiated by heparin.

Fig. 6.13 Features of heparin and warfarin

	Heparin (unfractionated)	Warfarin
Site of action	Potentiates antithrombin III	Inhibits vitamin K reductase
Route of administration	Subcutaneous/intravenous	Oral
Prothrombin time	Mildly prolonged	Prolonged
Activated partial thromboplastin time	Prolonged	Prolonged
Thrombin time	Prolonged	Normal

Anticoagulation

The main use of anticoagulants is to prevent unwanted thrombus formation or extension. They act on the clotting cascade to prevent fibrin formation. Anticoagulants do not prevent platelet plug formation, nor do they break down those which are already formed.

There are two commonly used anticoagulants: heparin and warfarin. A table summarizing the attributes of heparin and warfarin is given in Fig. 6.13. The type of anticoagulant and the duration of its use will depend on the indication for treatment. Indications for anticoagulation therapy include:

- Prophylaxis: mechanical prosthetic heart valves, atrial fibrillation, following surgery, unstable angina
- Post-thromboembolic event: deep vein thrombosis, pulmonary embolism, acute peripheral arterial occlusion, management of myocardial infarction
- During therapeutic procedures: cardiopulmonary bypass, haemodialysis.

The danger of using anticoagulants is the risk of haemorrhage. Patients already at risk of bleeding, e.g. those with peptic ulcers, oesophageal varices or severe hypertension, are contraindicated for anticoagulation. People given anticoagulants should be monitored closely to ensure the correct dose is being administered.

Warfarin

Warfarin is a vitamin K antagonist and will therefore reduce the activity of vitamin-K-dependent factors. It affects the factors in the order VII, IX, X and II due to their half-lives. Proteins C and S are also inacti-

Fig. 6.14 Target international normalized ratio (INR) for different indications of warfarin therapy

Indication	Target INR
DVT prophylaxis	2.5
Treatment of DVT/PE	2.5
Recurrent DVT/PE (on warfarin)	3.5
Atrial fibrillation	2.5
Dilated cardiomyopathy	2.5
Mural thrombus post MI	2.5
Rheumatic mitral valve disease	2.5
Mechanical heart valve	3.5

All targets are ±0.5. DVT, deep vein thrombosis; MI, myocardial infarction; PE, pulmonary embolus.

vated by warfarin. This occurs before thrombin inactivation causing a relative deficiency in proteins C and S, which can lead to skin necrosis due to extensive thrombosis of the microvasculature within the subcutaneous fat. Because warfarin acts primarily on the extrinsic pathway, the prothrombin time is used to monitor the effect on clotting (given as INR). The target INR for different indications is given in Fig. 6.14.

Care must be taken when using warfarin. It is teratogenic and therefore should not be used in early pregnancy (heparin does not cross the placenta and so can be used in pregnancy). Warfarin interacts with many drugs. Common interactions are shown in Fig. 6.15. Warfarin is potentiated in liver disease. Because warfarin has a half-life of 40 hours, the effects of changes in dose can take 4–5 days to become evident. If there is a warfarin overdose, i.e. the INR exceeds 4.5, warfarin should be

Fig. 6.15 Common drug interactions with warfarin

Increase anticoagulant effect	Decrease anticoagulant effect
Sulphonamides	Barbiturates
Metronidazole	Rifampicin
Cephalosporins	Oral contraceptives
Tricyclic antidepressants	Antifungals
Thyroxine	Antiepileptics (e.g.
Amiodarone	carbamazepine)
High-dose salicylates (aspirin)	
Excess paracetamol	
Alcohol	

stopped for 1 or 2 days and recommenced at a lower dose. The specific antidote to warfarin is vitamin K, which can be administered orally or intravenously. If the overdose has resulted in severe bleeding, fresh-frozen plasma or factor concentrates might be needed.

Heparin

Heparin is a glycosaminoglycan that potentiates the actions of ATIII. Standard (unfractionated) heparin contains molecules ranging in weight from 5000 to 30,000 kDa. The different chain lengths affect both activity and clearance, with the larger molecules being cleared more quickly. The activated partial thromboplastin time (APTT) is used to monitor unfractionated heparin therapy. Low-molecular-weight heparin (LMWH) has a mean molecular weight of 5000 kDa. LMWH is monitored only in renal failure and pregnancy. Monitoring is with an anti-Xa assay. LMWH differs from standard heparin because:

- It has greater activity against FXa than thrombin
- It has reduced protein binding and clearance
- Interactions with platelets are reduced.

LMWHs are commonly used, as subcutaneous injection, in the acute management of deep vein thrombosis (DVT) and pulmonary embolism (PE). Warfarin therapy is often started within 2 days and heparin stopped when the INR is >2.0. LMWH is the anticoagulant of choice for prophylaxis against venous thrombosis following surgery and is increasingly used as a prophylactic against DVT in non-surgical patients.

Long-term unfractionated heparin therapy can result in osteoporosis. Other complications include bleeding and heparin induced thrombocytopenia (HIT) which is a rare but serious problem. The risk of complications is less for LMWH than for unfractionated heparin.

Fibrinolysis

In blood, the fibrinolytic system breaks down excessive thrombus formation in the lumen of the vessels, thus preventing luminal occlusion. Plasminogen is activated, by cleaving an arginine–valine bond, to form plasmin. Activation can be intrinsic (by FXIIa or kallikrein) or extrinsic (by tissue plasminogen activator (tPA) or by urokinase). Many mechanisms, e.g. thrombin-activated fibrinolysis inhibitor, plasminogen activator inhibitor, α_2-antiplasmin, closely regulate fibrinolysis.

Tissue plasminogen activator

tPA is released from activated endothelial cells and is the most important activator of fibrinolysis. It binds to fibrin, where it activates plasminogen that is already bound to the thrombus. This ensures that plasmin production is localized to the clot. Inhibitors of tPA are destroyed by protein C, enhancing fibrinolysis.

Plasmin

Plasmin cleaves peptide bonds in fibrin to produce degradation products of various sizes. Small fragments, termed 'D' fragments, are produced in large quantities in conditions such as disseminated intravascular coagulation (see p. 123). D-dimers can be detected in the plasma or urine using a diagnostic test.

Therapeutic fibrinolysis

Fibrinolytic agents are used in life-threatening venous thrombosis, pulmonary embolism, myocardial infarction and stroke. They attempt to restore blood supply to an area of the circulation that has been occluded by a fibrin clot. There are different fibrinolytic agents available:

- Streptokinase: derived from group A β-haemolytic streptococci. It binds to plasminogen to form a complex that can activate other plasminogen molecules. It is highly antigenic

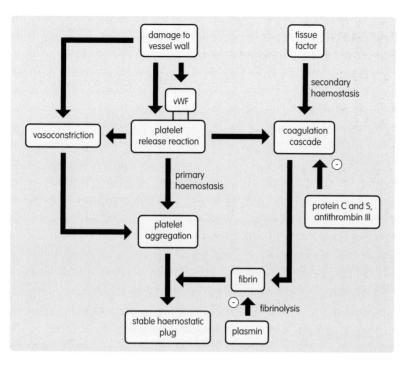

Fig. 6.16 Overview of haemostasis. vWF, von Willebrand's factor.

- Urokinase: derived from human kidney cells. It is a tPA originally isolated in urine
- Recombinant tPA: synthesized from human cells. It is highly specific for plasminogen and has a short half-life of 2–6 minutes.

Overview of haemostasis

The role of platelets, the clotting cascade and fibrinolysis in haemostasis are outlined in Fig. 6.16.

Bleeding disorders that result from a clotting defect or thrombocytopenia can be distinguished by their clinical features. Patients with haemophilia present with bleeding deep in tissues whereas patients with thrombocytopenia present with superficial bleeding into the skin or mucous membranes.

CLOTTING FACTOR DISORDERS

Clotting factor abnormalities can be hereditary or acquired.

Hereditary factor abnormalities
von Willebrand's disease

von Willebrand's disease, a deficiency or defect in von Willebrand's factor (vWF), is the most common hereditary bleeding disorder, affecting perhaps as many as 1% of the population. vWF is the carrier protein for FVIII in plasma, and stabilizes it, prolonging its survival in the circulation. It also promotes platelet interactions. There are several types of the disease:

- Type 1: partial deficiency of circulating normal vWF molecules
- Type 2A: absence of the largest vWF multimers
- Type 2B: synthesis of abnormal vWF multimers
- Type 2M: defective GPIb binding site
- Type 2N: reduced affinity for FVIII
- Type 3: absolute deficiency of circulating vWF.

Type 1 is the most common form of the disease. Impaired release of normally synthesized vWF multimers from endothelial cells leads to a deficiency of vWF. This can be partially corrected by an infusion of arginine vasopressin.

The severity of clinical symptoms is very variable in type 1 and is usually more severe in type 2. The impairment of platelet adhesion and FVIII deficiency can cause mucous membrane bleeding and excessive blood loss following injuries and surgery. In type 3 disease, which is a rare severe bleeding disorder, there may be spontaneous bleeds into muscles and joints.

Haemophilia A

Haemophilia A is caused by a deficiency of FVIII. The prevalence of haemophilia A in males is 1 in 5000 and is not affected by geographic, ethnic or religious association, or by social class. Haemophilia A is an X-linked recessive condition, therefore overwhelmingly affecting males. In 33% of all haemophilia A cases, patients have no family history of the disease and such cases are thought to arise from spontaneous mutation of the FVIII gene. The normal plasma concentration of FVIII ranges from 0.5 to 2 IU/mL. The frequency and severity of bleeding correlates with the plasma level of FVIII. Haemophilia A can be classified as severe, moderate or mild (Fig. 6.17) with severe disease accounting for ~70% of haemophilic patients.

> The most common clinical feature of haemophilia is bleeding into joints (haemarthrosis); muscular bleeding is the next most common and together they make up 95% of how patients with severe haemophilia present. Other possible presenting symptoms include nose bleeds, GI bleeding, haematuria and prolonged bleeding following surgery or dental extraction.
>
> Some of the most serious consequences of bleeds include:
> - Chronic damage: fixed flexion deformities of the limbs with muscle atrophy, neurological damage
> - Acute problems: compartment syndrome, compression of the respiratory tract, massive loss of circulating volume and intracranial haemorrhage.

Factor replacement therapy

Factor VIII can be replaced with:

- Recombinant FVIII
- Plasma-derived FVIII concentrates.

These can be infused following injury to raise the level of FVIII to between 30% and 100% of normal. Prophylactic treatment with FVIII is currently recommended in children with severe haemophilia.

Fig. 6.17 Symptoms of haemophilia A

Concentration of coagulation factor (% of normal)	Bleeding episodes
50–100	None
25–50	Bleeding tendency after severe trauma
5–25 Mild	Severe bleeding episodes after surgery, slight bleeding episodes after minor trauma
1–5 Moderate	Severe bleeding episodes even after slight trauma
<1 Severe	Spontaneous bleeding episodes predominantly in the joints or muscles

The baseline of FVIII is raised above 2%, converting 'severe' to 'moderate' disease.

There is a risk of iatrogenic infections from all blood products. Haemophiliacs, not treated with recombinant products, are exposed to blood products from many donors (pooled plasma is used to concentrate FVIII) on many occasions each year (average 31 bleeding episodes per year). Over 50% of haemophiliacs in the USA and Europe contracted HIV from infected blood products before screening for HIV was introduced; many also contracted hepatitis C. AIDS has been a common cause of death in haemophiliacs, with many also developing chronic hepatitis and cirrhosis. In the UK the recombinant product is recommended.

Haemophilia B

Haemophilia B (Christmas disease), caused by a deficiency of FIX, is also X-linked. Haemophilia A and B can be differentiated only by specific coagulation factor assays. Haemophilia B has an identical pattern of clinical features to haemophilia A, but is five times less common. Treatment is similar to that for haemophilia A, but with FIX replacement rather than FVIII. FIX has a longer half-life than FVIII and therefore fewer infusions are required.

A normal PT with an abnormal APPT is suggestive of haemophilia.

Fig. 6.18 Overview of the major hereditary clotting factor deficiencies

Feature	Haemophilia A	Haemophilia B	von Willebrand's disease
Deficiency	Factor VIII	Factor IX	vWF and moderate reduction in factor VIII
Inheritance	X-linked	X-linked	Commonly autosomal dominant with incomplete penetration
Main sites of bleeding	Muscles, joints, post-trauma/surgery	Muscles, joints, post-trauma/surgery	Mucous membranes, skin cuts, post-trauma/surgery, menorrhagia
Platelet count	Normal	Normal	Normal
Platelet aggregation	Normal	Normal	Impaired
Bleeding time	Normal	Normal	Prolonged
Prothrombin time	Normal	Normal	Normal
APTT	Prolonged	Prolonged	Prolonged or normal

APTT, activated partial thromboplastin time; vWF, von Willebrand's factor.

Other deficiencies

Hereditary deficiencies of the other coagulation factors are rare. As in haemophilias A and B, the severity of the disorders is related to the degree of deficiency. In specific areas, the prevalence of a certain coagulation factor deficiency can be much higher than average. Examples of this are a high prevalence of FVII deficiency in Northern Italy and a high prevalence of FXI deficiency among Ashkenazi Jews.

Fig. 6.18 shows a summary of hereditary factor deficiencies.

Acquired factor abnormalities
Vitamin K deficiency

Vitamin K deficiency is discussed on page 119.

Liver disease

The liver produces all the clotting factors except for vWF; liver disease is therefore associated with clotting factor deficiency. In addition, biliary obstruction can lead to malabsorption and deficiency of fat-soluble vitamin K. This leads to decreased synthesis of the vitamin-K-dependent factors. Portal hypertension can lead to splenomegaly, resulting in increased splenic sequestration of platelets. In severe liver disease, levels of FV and fibrinogen are reduced, and increased levels of plasminogen activator are present. An acquired dysfibrinogenaemia (functional abnormality of fibrinogen) is also seen in many patients.

Disseminated intravascular coagulation (DIC)

DIC arises from excessive activation of the coagulation cascade, followed by activation of the fibrinolytic system. Coagulation is activated in two ways:

1. Release of tissue factor from damaged tissues, monocytes or red blood cells
2. Activation of factors XI and XII by damaged vascular endothelium.

There is generalized fibrin deposition on vascular endothelium, with extensive consumption of platelets and coagulation factors. Small vessels are obstructed, leading to tissue damage and multiple organ dysfunction.

Fibrin deposition activates the fibrinolytic pathway and results in the formation of fibrin degradation products (FDPs). FDPs inhibit fibrin polymerization and consequently impair coagulation. The net result is a bleeding disorder due to a lack of platelets and clotting factors, and inhibition of fibrin polymerization by FDPs. In DIC, PT, APTT and thrombin clotting times can all be prolonged.

Causes of DIC include:

- Acute: obstetric complications, septicaemia, acute haemolysis, shock
- Subacute: malignancy
- Chronic: liver disease, malignancy.

The management of DIC involves treatment of the underlying disorder and supportive care with transfusion of fresh frozen plasma, cryoprecipitate and platelets.

THROMBOSIS

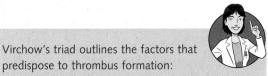

Virchow's triad outlines the factors that predispose to thrombus formation:
- Changes in blood flow
- Changes in blood constituents
- Changes within the walls of blood vessels.

Venous thromboembolism (VTE)

Thrombosis is the formation of a blood clot (thrombus) in the circulation from blood constituents; an embolism is the occlusion of a vessel by foreign material or a blood clot (thromboembolism) which has moved from its starting position.

Deep vein thrombosis (DVT) occurs most commonly in the lower limbs. Symptoms and signs include:
- Swelling (usually asymmetrical)
- Pain (especially on dorsiflexion)
- Erythema.

If part of a DVT dislodges to form an embolus, this can lodge in the vasculature of the lung, a so-called pulmonary embolism (PE). PE can present most severely as collapse but symptoms often include:
- Dyspnoea
- Tachypnoea
- Pleuritic chest pain.

Well's criteria are used to evaluate the probability of VTE. A normal D-dimer level is useful to exclude VTE but may be raised in many conditions. Doppler ultrasound is used to diagnose thrombosis and a V/Q scan or spiral CT for PE.

Virchow's triad provides a framework to think about the risk factors for VTE formation.

Hypercoagulability

Thrombophilias are disorders of haemostasis that increase the tendency of blood to clot. These may be inherited or acquired.

Primary (hereditary) thrombophilia

Antithrombin III deficiency

ATIII deficiency is an autosomal dominant condition affecting 1 in 2000 people. The deficiency is either:

- Type I (decreased quantity)
- Type II (reduced biological activity).

Heterozygotes have 40–50% of normal plasma ATIII levels; homozygosity is lethal. Most patients with ATIII deficiency experience a thrombotic episode before the age of 50 years. Thrombosis might be severe and recurrent and these patients might have to have their blood anticoagulated with warfarin long term (see also p. 119).

Deficiencies of proteins C and S

Inheritance for both protein C and protein S deficiencies is autosomal dominant. Protein S deficiency is clinically indistinguishable from protein C deficiency. As with ATIII deficiency, they can be type I (decreased quantity) or type II (reduced biological activity). Heterozygotes have 50% of normal levels of protein C or S. Clinical features are similar to ATIII deficiency, but the thrombotic risk is four times lower. Homozygous protein C deficiency has been described where individuals have less than 1% of normal levels of protein C and have very severe disease, often presenting with problems at birth. Because proteins C and S have a shorter half-life than vitamin-K-dependent factors II, IX and X, warfarin therapy causes a temporary prothrombotic state and can lead to skin necrosis.

Defective fibrinolysis

Abnormal plasminogen and fibrinogen have been associated with reduced fibrinolytic activity and a tendency of blood to clot.

Activated protein C resistance due to factor V Leiden

A missense mutation of the FV gene (arginine is replaced by glutamine) renders FV ten times less sensitive to inactivation by activated protein C. This disorder has an incidence in Caucasians in the UK of 5% and might account for the majority of cases of inherited thrombophilia. This mutation acts as a cofactor in the following hypercoagulable states:

- Oral contraceptive pill and pregnancy
- Surgery and immobility
- Other thrombophilia disorders.

Prothrombin allele G20210A

Between 2% and 3% of the population have this prothrombin variant, which increases prothrombin levels and the thrombotic risk.

Hyperhomocysteinaemia

High levels of plasma homocysteine increase the risk of venous and arterial thrombosis.

Secondary (acquired) thrombophilia

The following conditions are associated with an increased incidence of thrombosis:

- Prolonged immobilization of the patient (venous stasis)
- Disseminated cancer (secretion of tumour substances that activate FX)
- Oestrogen therapy (increased plasma levels of factors II, VII, IX and X, and reduced levels of ATIII and tPA)
- Myeloproliferative disorders
- Sickle-cell anaemia

- The antiphospholipid antibody syndrome (lupus anticoagulant syndrome). This disorder is characterized by the presence of antiphospholipid antibodies in association with a clinical event. The main features of this syndrome are arterial or venous thrombosis or complications in pregnancy such as recurrent miscarriage. The disease can be idiopathic or secondary to other autoimmune disorders such as SLE.

Endothelial injury

Factors such as smoking, hypercholesterolaemia, hypertension, infection and immune-mediated damage contribute to endothelial injury and subsequent thrombus formation.

Alterations to blood flow

In conditions such as atrial fibrillation, where the flow of blood is altered, a thrombus can be formed within the circulation.

INDICATIONS FOR BLOOD TRANSFUSION

Indications for blood transfusion include:

- Trauma
- Surgery
- Shock
- Severe anaemia, e.g. that associated with haemoglobinopathies.

Some individuals do not wish to receive another person's blood, either as a result of religious beliefs or because they wish to avoid the risks associated with blood transfusion. The alternatives to blood transfusion include:

- Volume expanders: used in the acute setting to avoid the onset of shock
- Growth factors (EPO): are not used in the acute situation; they work by stimulating the bone marrow to produce more RBCs
- Intraoperative blood salvage: blood lost during surgery is collected and reinfused into the patient
- Autologous blood donation: an individual donates their own blood that can be saved and infused back into the individual should they need it. This has been used for fit patients having planned surgery. Cheating athletes sometimes use this to aid their performance, a process called blood doping, as it is hard to test for
- Synthetic blood substitutes: have not yet been fully achieved; haemoglobin-based oxygen carriers and perfluorochemical compounds can perform some red cell function, but nothing has been developed yet to fully replace blood.

The main concern when administering a blood transfusion is the avoidance of an adverse immunological reaction as a result of an incompatibility between donor and recipient blood. Adverse immunological reactions occur because there are a variety of antigens on the surface of red cells. Thus, when an individual is exposed to red blood cells with different antibodies (to which they are therefore not self-tolerant), they are attacked by the immune system.

RED-CELL ANTIGENS

The surfaces of red cells are covered with antigenic molecules. Over 400 different groups of antigens have been identified, although only some of these are clinically important in blood transfusion. Some red-cell antigens can be recognized by antibodies in the serum of a recipient of a blood transfusion and can cause an adverse reaction. These reactions can be severe and life threatening, so it is important to identify the antigens and antibodies present in both donor and recipient blood.

ABO antigens

The ABO system consists of three allelic genes, A, B and O, which code for sugar-residue transferase enzymes. The ABO antigen, known as the H antigen, is a glycoprotein or glycolipid with a terminal L-fructose.

Fig. 7.1 ABO antigens. *N*-acgal, *N*-acetyl galactosamine; gal, galactose.

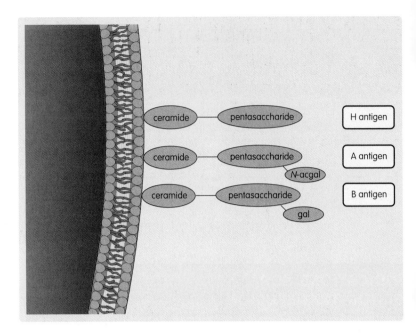

ceramide — pentasaccharide — H antigen

ceramide — pentasaccharide — A antigen
N-acgal

ceramide — pentasaccharide — B antigen
gal

Fig. 7.2 ABO blood groups

Phenotype/red-cell antigens	Genotype	Antibodies
O	OO	Anti-A and anti-B
A	AO or AA	Anti-B
B	BO or BB	Anti-A
AB	AB	None

- The O gene is amorphous, i.e. it has no effect on antigenic structure and leaves antigen H unchanged
- The group A gene product adds *N*-acetyl galactosamine to the H antigen
- The group B gene product adds the sugar D-galactose (Fig. 7.1).

Inheritance of the three ABO alleles can lead to six different genotypes and four possible phenotypes (Fig. 7.2).

By 6 months of age, the immune system will have been exposed to A- and B-like antigens in intestinal bacteria and food substances. IgM antibodies develop against A and/or B antigens, unless these antigens are present on red cells (self-tolerance). Transfused blood must be ABO-compatible with the recipient's blood, otherwise recipient antibody will cause agglutination and haemolysis of the transfused cells. For example, if group A red cells are given to a group O recipient, anti-A antibodies in the recipient's serum will destroy the donor cells.

Ideally, ABO-identical blood is used; however, if this is not possible, compatible blood can be used. Blood cells of group O are not affected by anti-A or anti-B antibodies and can therefore be given to patients of any blood group. Consequently, blood group O is referred to as the universal donor, although it should be borne in mind that the serum of individuals with group O blood will contain anti-A and anti-B antibodies. It is always more desirable to use group-specific red cells for transfusion. Conversely, AB individuals are universal recipients because they do not possess anti-ABO antibodies and can receive blood of any ABO type.

Rhesus antigens

Rhesus (Rh) antigens are good immunogens and the antibodies generated are clinically important. They are known as C, D and E, but the D antigen is the most important clinically; it is the D antigen that is referred to when describing someone as 'rhesus positive' or 'rhesus negative'. The rhesus locus on chromosome 1 consists of two closely linked genes, RhD and RhCE, which are inherited together. RhD

Fig. 7.3 Rhesus genotypes

CDE genotype	RhD
cde/cde	Negative
CDe/cde	Positive
CDe/CDe	Positive
cDE/cde	Positive
CDe/cDE	Positive
cDE/cDE	Positive
Others	Most are positive

encodes the D antigen; 'd' denotes the absence of D antigen (Fig. 7.3). The gene RhCE encodes antigens named C, c, E and e. Note that 'c' and 'e' are real antigens and not just the absence of an antigen, like 'd'. Alternate gene splicing of RhCE produces two proteins.

D antigen is the strongest immunogen. Rh positive individuals are DD or Dd, Rh negative individuals are dd. Approximately 85% of Caucasians are Rh positive and 15% are Rh negative.

Anti-D antibodies are only generated when an Rh negative individual is exposed to Rh positive red cells following transfusion or pregnancy. All anti-D antibodies are IgG. Approximately 70% of Rh negative individuals produce anti-D antibodies after receiving Rh positive blood and they will develop transfusion reactions when re-transfused with Rh positive blood.

In an emergency, if there is no time to cross-match blood, O negative is given.

RhD haemolytic disease of the newborn

If blood from an Rh positive fetus enters the circulation of an Rh negative mother, alloimmunization can occur. Small amounts of fetal blood are transferred during the third trimester and at birth. Mothers develop anti-D IgG antibodies, which cross the placenta into the fetal circulation during the course of the second pregnancy. If the second fetus is Rh positive, the IgG antibodies induce immune haemolysis of fetal red cells, which can result in hydrops fetalis.

Prevention of RhD haemolytic disease of the newborn

Passive immunization is utilized to prevent maternal anti-D antibody production. The mother is given an intramuscular injection of anti-D IgG at 28 weeks and within 72 hours of the birth. The injected antibody coats Rh positive fetal red blood cells, which are removed by the reticuloendothelial system (RES) before the mother produces her own anti-D antibodies. The dose of anti-D IgG can be adjusted depending on the volume of fetal red blood cells in the maternal circulation, as estimated by the Kleihauer technique. Anti-D antibody is also used following abortion in Rh negative women and following transfusion of Rh positive blood into Rh negative individuals.

Red-cell antigens other than rhesus D, such as Kell and ABO incompatibility, can also cause haemolytic disease of the newborn. Although ABO incompatibility leading to haemolytic disease of the newborn may occur during the first pregnancy, therapy should be given during every pregnancy to avoid problems.

Other red-cell antigens

Other red-cell antigens include:

- P
- Lewis
- I
- MN
- Kell
- Duffy
- Kidd.

CROSS-MATCHING AND BLOOD TRANSFUSION

Cross-matching blood

It is important to correctly identify the patient and to label samples accurately before blood transfusions to prevent potentially fatal transfusion reactions. Cross-matching has three stages:

1. Blood grouping (ABO and Rh) of the recipient
2. Screening for abnormal recipient antibodies
   - indirect antiglobulin test: the recipient's serum is tested against a standard pool of red cells to detect antibodies to blood group antigens other than those of the ABO and Rh systems
   - screening cells and cell panels
3. Each unit of donor blood to be transfused is then tested against the patient's serum to identify atypical antibodies.

Emergency transfusions

Patients requiring emergency transfusions, e.g. for acute haemorrhage, should receive plasma-depleted red cells. Red cells are suspended in SAG-M (saline–adenine–glucose–mannitol—a nutrient solution). This contains little plasma and therefore reduces the risk of transfusing blood group antibodies or proteins. Patients can be issued with group-specific red cells that have not been cross-matched if time is of the essence. Flying squads are issued with O negative which has not been crossed-matched.

Filtering and warming at transfusion

Blood giving sets with filters are no longer an absolute requirement for leucodepletion as donor blood is leucodepleted at the transfusion centre; however, filters are still used to help avoid contamination. Blood is warmed when it is rapidly transfused to prevent vasoconstriction, which would reduce the rate of transfusion.

Dangers in the use of blood products

Transfusion reaction

Transfusion reactions occur when incompatible blood is transfused. A summary of the complications of blood transfusions is given in Fig. 7.4.

Haemolytic transfusion reactions

Haemolytic transfusion reaction

Haemolytic transfusion reactions are the most serious complication of blood transfusion and usually occur as a result of ABO incompatibility. Intravascular haemolysis occurs through the activation of complement with IgM, causing symptoms of:
- Dyspnoea
- Rigors
- Lumbar pain
- Flushing
- Urticaria
- Headache.

If blood is noticed in the urine, kidney failure is of immediate concern.

Release of vasoactive substances causes profound hypotension and shock, and renal tubular necrosis can cause acute renal failure. Release of tissue thromboplastin from lysed red cells can lead to disseminated intravascular coagulation (DIC). Death occurs in 15% of cases of ABO incompatibility and usually results from severe DIC or renal failure.

Extravascular haemolysis, mediated by IgG, occurs more slowly and is less severe.

Fig. 7.4 Complications of blood transfusions	
Early	**Late**
Haemolytic reactions (immediate/delayed)	Transfusion transmitted infection:
Allergic reactions to white cells, platelets or proteins (e.g. urticaria, anaphylaxis)	• Viral (e.g. CMV, HIV, hepatitis)
Febrile reactions	• Bacterial (e.g. Salmonella)
Transfusion-related acute lung injury	• Parasites (e.g. malaria, Toxoplasma)
Circulatory overload	Iron overload
Air embolism	Alloimmunization (might cause rhesus haemolytic disease in the future)
Thrombophlebitis	Graft-versus-host disease
Hyperkalaemia	
Clotting abnormalities	

CMV, cytomegalovirus; HIV, human immunodeficiency virus.

The most severe transfusion reaction, acute haemolysis, is caused by the destruction of donor red blood cells by antibodies (IgG or IgM) present in the recipient's serum. Haemolysis caused by IgM occurs immediately, reactions caused by IgG are delayed:

- Extravascular haemolysis results from incompatibilities of blood groups that produce IgG antibodies, e.g. Rh, Kell, Duffy and Kidd. Antibody-coated red blood cells are then removed by the RES
- ABO incompatibility (usually due to a clerical error) causes intravascular haemolysis when IgM antibodies fix complement. Activation of complement generates C3a and C5a, which cause vasodilatation, increased vascular permeability and neutrophil chemotaxis.

Blood products and infection risk

Infections have been transmitted in blood products. To minimize infection risk, donor blood is screened for several infective agents including syphilis, hepatitis B and C, and HIV.

Detection techniques are not foolproof. For example, HIV is detected by the presence of antibodies in donor blood. HIV has been transmitted in blood products from donors who had not seroconverted at the time of donation. Blood is taken aseptically and is then leucodepleted to reduce the risk of transmission.

There is concern about the transmission of variant Creutzfeldt–Jakob disease (vCJD), with reported cases of presumed transmission of vCJD in blood products. For this reason British plasma is no longer used in the treatment of congenital bleeding disorders.

Iron overload

The levels of iron in the body are usually controlled by the regulation of absorption. There are no physiological mechanisms to eliminate iron from the body. When people receive multiple blood transfusions, the excess iron is deposited in, and causes damage to, the heart, liver and endocrine organs. Iron-chelating agents, such as desferrioxamine and deferiprone, facilitate iron excretion.

Other blood products

Platelets

Platelets are stored at room temperature (on an oscillating tray to prevent clumping) and have a half-life of 4–5 days. They can be obtained from a pool of 6–10 blood donors or from a single donor via apheresis. Indications for platelet transfusion include:

- Patients who are bleeding and who have a platelet count $<50 \times 10^9/L$
- Following massive transfusion resulting in dilutional thrombocytopenia
- Patients with platelet dysfunction who are bleeding
- Prophylactically in patients with thrombocytopenia who are undergoing surgery or who have bone marrow failure.

Apheresis

Apheresis allows the removal of one specific component of blood such as platelets. Blood withdrawn is separated and the selected component taken out. The rest of the blood is then returned to the donor. The time this takes depends on the blood component required and is usually in the region of 1–2 hours.

Importantly, since most of the blood taken is returned, a large amount of the select component can be taken. This means that the recipient is exposed to products from fewer donors and thus the chance of adverse reactions and infections.

Fresh-frozen plasma

Fresh-frozen plasma (FFP) contains albumin, immunoglobulins and all the clotting factors. Indications for FFP transfusion include:

- Multiple clotting factor deficiencies, e.g. severe liver disease, warfarin overdose, massive transfusion (more than 10 units within 24 hours) and thrombotic thrombocytopenic purpura where it is used in plasma exchange
- Specific coagulation factor replacement where no concentrate is available
- Plasma loss (albumin solution is used in many cases, e.g. burns).

Compatibility of plasma is the opposite of red cells, e.g. O plasma contains anti-A and anti-B antibodies so it should only be given to O recipients.

Cryoprecipitate

Cryoprecipitate is the insoluble precipitate formed when FFP is thawed at 4°C. It contains factors VIII, vWF, factor XIII and fibrinogen, and is given to control bleeding associated with defects thereof. Cryoprecipitate can also be of use in chronic renal failure, advanced liver failure, disseminated intravascular coagulation and following massive blood transfusion.

Clotting factor concentrates

Specific clotting factor concentrates can be given to patients with clotting factor deficiencies (see Chapter 6).

White cells

Granulocyte concentrates can be given to infected neutropenic patients not responding to antibiotic therapy, but this is rare because of the risk of cytomegalovirus (CMV) transmission.

Haematological investigations

You should be able to:
- Understand how and when the following investigations are performed:
  - Full blood count
  - Differential white count
  - Peripheral blood film
  - Electrophoresis
  - Bone marrow investigations
  - Lymph node biopsy
  - Cytogenetic analysis
  - Erythrocyte sedimentation rate (ESR)
  - Clotting tests
- Recognize the different blood cells present on a blood film.

Normal ranges can vary with each laboratory. It is therefore important to check the normal ranges from the lab which the blood results you are looking at come from. The normal range is usually printed close to the result.

FULL BLOOD COUNT AND RETICULOCYTE COUNT

Blood samples are added to EDTA, an anticoagulant. The samples are tested by an automated analyser, which provides the following information:

- Hb concentration, haematocrit, red-cell count, mean cell volume (MCV) and mean cell haemoglobin (MCH)
- White-cell count with differential
- Platelet count: some laboratories produce additional parameters
- RDW (red cell distribution width): a measure of the range of red blood cell size in a sample.

Red-cell parameters and the diagnostic inferences of abnormalities of the full blood count are shown in Fig. 8.1.

DIFFERENTIAL WHITE COUNT

The differential white count breaks down the white-cell count to identify the level of each of the five peripheral white cell lines: neutrophils, lymphocytes, monocytes, eosinophils and basophils. This is automated and uses stains, cell size and light scatter to differentiate between the different cells. The parameters for white cells and platelets, and the diagnostic inferences made from their abnormalities, are given in Fig. 8.2.

PERIPHERAL BLOOD FILM

Examination of a peripheral blood film is a simple haematological investigation, which can provide a significant amount of information. Blood is evenly spread into a film on a glass slide, which is then dried and stained, most often with a Romanowsky stain. The peripheral blood film shows the morphology of blood cells and can show inclusions within the cells. Abnormalities of red and white cells that are identified on the peripheral blood film are shown in Figs 8.3 and 8.4, respectively.

Normal blood cells

Normal peripheral blood films are shown in Figs 8.5–8.11.

Fig. 8.1 Red-cell parameters on peripheral full blood count

Parameter	Normal range		Diagnostic inference of abnormalities
	Male	Female	
Red-cell count	$4.4–5.8 \times 10^{12}$/L	$4.0–5.2 \times 10^{12}$/L	
Haemoglobin Packed cell volume or haematocrit	13–17 g/dL 40–51%	12–15 g/dL 38–48%	↑ Polycythaemia ↓ Anaemia
Mean cell volume	80–100 fL		↑ (macrocytic) Vitamin B_{12} or folate deficiency, pregnancy, neonates, alcohol or chronic liver disease (may be haemolysis or aplastic anaemia) ↓ (microcytic) Iron deficiency, thalassaemia or anaemia of chronic disease
Mean cell haemoglobin	27–32 pg		↓ (hypochromic) Occurs with microcytosis
Mean cell haemoglobin concentration	32–36 g/dL		
Reticulocyte count	1–2% of circulating red cells $10–100 \times 10^9$/L		↑ (reticulocytosis) Haemolytic anaemias and after acute blood loss ↓ (reticulocytopenia) Impaired red-cell production

Packed cell volume, otherwise known as the haematocrit, is equal to the red-cell count multiplied by the mean cell volume. Mean cell haemoglobin is the haemoglobin divided by the red-cell count, while the mean cell haemoglobin concentration is the haemoglobin divided by the haematocrit. Automated analysers are increasingly able to carry out reticulocyte counts, although they are also carried out on peripheral blood films stained with new methylene blue. The normal range represents values for 95% of the population (mean ±2 standard deviations).

Fig. 8.2 The differential white-cell count and its abnormalities

Parameters	Normal range	Diagnostic inference
White cell count	$4–11 \times 10^9$/L	↑ (leucocytosis); ↓ (leucopenia)
Neutrophils	$2–7.5 \times 10^9$/L (40–80%)	↑ (neutrophilia); ↓ (neutropenia)
Lymphocytes	$1.3–3.5 \times 10^9$/L (20–40%)	↑ (lymphocytosis); ↓ (lymphopenia)
Monocytes	$0.2–0.8 \times 10^9$/L (2–10%)	↑ (monocytosis)
Eosinophils	$0.04–0.44 \times 10^9$/L (1–6%)	↑ (eosinophilia)
Basophils	$0–0.1 \times 10^9$/L (<1–2%)	↑ (basophilia)
Platelet count	$150–400 \times 10^9$/L	↑ Reactive (thrombocytosis): haemorrhage, infection, malignancy, inflammation; or pathological (thrombocythaemia); myeloproliferative disorders ↓ (thrombocytopenia)

Percentages given indicate the normal percentage of the white-cell count. Abnormalities of white cells can be seen in Chapter 5, thrombocytopenia is covered in Chapter 6. The normal range represents values for 95% of the population (mean ±2 standard deviations).

Fig. 8.3 Red cell abnormalities on the peripheral blood film

Abnormality	Description	Diagnostic inferences
Anisocytosis	Increased variation in size	See causes of micro- and macrocytosis in Fig. 8.1
Poikilocytosis	Increased variation in shape	Certain shapes are diagnostic for certain conditions
Spherocytes	Small spherical cells lacking central pallor	Hereditary spherocytosis, warm AIHA
Sickle cells	Crescent-shaped cells	Sickle-cell anaemia
Target cells	Cells with central and peripheral dark-staining areas separated by a clear area	Thalassaemia syndromes, sickle-cell syndromes, iron deficiency, liver disease
Teardrop cells	Teardrop-shaped cells	Myelofibrosis, extramedullary haemopoiesis
Elliptocyte	Elliptical cell	Hereditary elliptocytosis
Echinocyte	Long projections from cell surface	Renal disease
Acanthocyte	Irregular outline	Liver disease, postsplenectomy, abetalipoproteinaemia
Fragments	Small red cell fragments	DIC, microangiopathy, cardiac valve replacement
Howell–Jolly bodies	Small nuclear inclusions normally removed by the spleen	Postsplenectomy, hyposplenism
Heinz bodies	Precipitates of oxidized denatured haemoglobin	Glucose-6-phosphate dehydrogenase deficiency
Hypochromia	Large area of central pallor	Reduced mean cell haemoglobin (see Fig. 8.1)
Polychromasia (recticulocytosis)	Large, bluish cells best seen on supravital staining with new methylene blue	See Fig. 8.1
Rouleaux	Red cell stacking (like piles of coins)	Multiple myeloma, Waldenström's macroglobulinaemia, any case with a high ESR

The normal red cell is normochromic, normocytic and has an area of central pallor. AIHA, autoimmune haemolytic anaemia; DIC, disseminated intravascular coagulation.

Fig. 8.4 White cell abnormalities on the peripheral blood film

Abnormality	Description	Diagnostic inferences
Hypersegmented neutrophils	Neutrophil nucleus containing >5 lobes	Megaloblastic anaemia
Left shift of myeloid cells	Immature myeloid cells, e.g. band cells, metamyelocytes	Pregnancy, severe infection, chronic myeloid leukaemia
Blast cells	Variable appearance	Acute myeloblastic or lymphoblastic leukaemia
Auer rods	Rod-like inclusions within the cytoplasm of leukaemic blasts and promyelocytes	Acute myeloblastic leukaemia
Smear cells	'Smudges' representing disrupted cells	Lymphocytosis—usually chronic lymphocytic leukaemia, but not always malignant
Leucoerythroblastic change	Nucleated red cells and immature leucocytes	Severe haemorrhage/haemolysis, bone marrow infiltration

Fig. 8.5 Normal red cells and platelets. Normal red cells are ~7.2 µm in diameter, and have a central pallor due to their biconcave shape. Platelets are seen on the film as small, irregular, densely staining cells (courtesy Professor Victor Hoffbrand and Dr John Pettit).

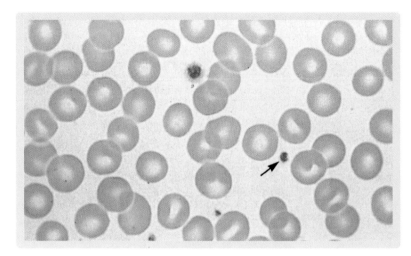

Fig. 8.6 Reticulocytes can be detected using supravital staining, which precipitates RNA in the cell. They are usually present in the blood in small numbers (courtesy Professor Victor Hoffbrand and Dr John Pettit).

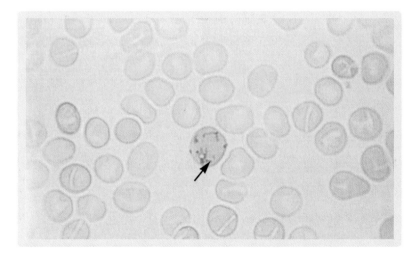

Fig. 8.7 Normal neutrophils have a characteristic multilobed nucleus (connected by chromatin). The cytoplasm is granular (courtesy Professor Victor Hoffbrand and Dr John Pettit).

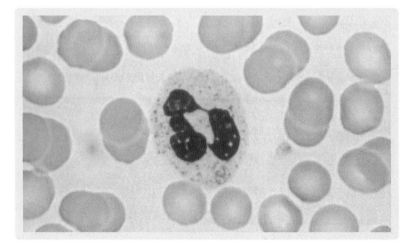

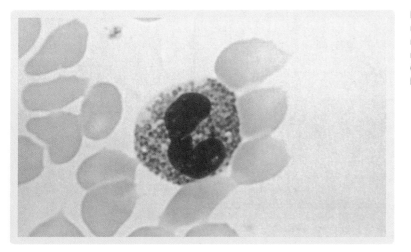

Fig. 8.8 Normal eosinophils are usually slightly larger than neutrophils. They have a bilobed nucleus and coarse granules (courtesy Professor Victor Hoffbrand and Dr John Pettit).

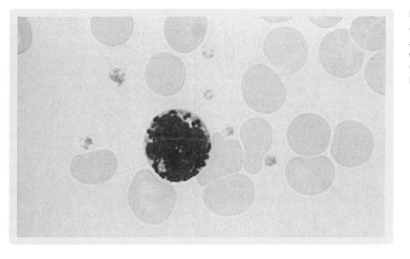

Fig. 8.9 Normal basophils contain a lobed nucleus with very coarse granules. They are the least common white cell in the blood (courtesy Professor Victor Hoffbrand and Dr John Pettit).

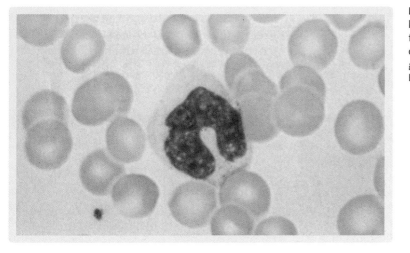

Fig. 8.10 Normal monocytes are large. The nucleus tends to be folded, not lobed, and the cytoplasm contains very fine granules (courtesy Professor Victor Hoffbrand and Dr John Pettit).

Fig. 8.11 Normal lymphocytes are quite small (9 μm diameter). They contain very little cytoplasm and occasional azurophilic granules (courtesy Professor Victor Hoffbrand and Dr John Pettit).

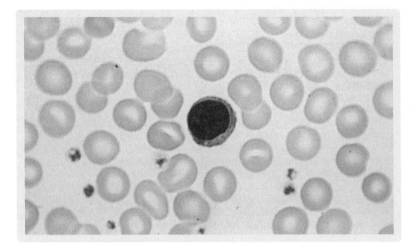

Fig. 8.12 Iron-deficiency anaemia. Red blood cells are typically hypochromic and microcytic (courtesy Professor Victor Hoffbrand and Dr John Pettit).

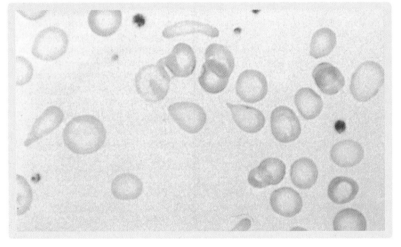

Peripheral blood films can be used in the diagnosis of haematological disease, for example:

- Iron-deficiency anaemia (Fig. 8.12)
- Hereditary spherocytosis (Fig. 8.13)
- Sickle-cell anaemia (Fig. 8.14)
- Multiple myeloma (Fig. 8.15).

The concept of right shift is illustrated in Fig. 8.16.

mixture, in which each of the molecules travels at a different rate, depending on its electrical charge and size. In terms of haemoglobinopathies, the different types of haemoglobin have different structures and therefore different weights/charges, so the pattern of bands produced by electrophoresis is different (Fig. 8.17).

INVESTIGATION OF HAEMOGLOBINOPATHIES

Electrophoresis

Electrophoresis is a method used to separate out biological molecules of similar size. An electric current is passed through a medium containing the

BONE MARROW INVESTIGATION

Bone marrow smear

Bone marrow smears allow examination of the stages of haemopoiesis. Bone marrow smears are usually stained with Romanowsky dyes, but Perls' Prussian blue may be used to detect iron in

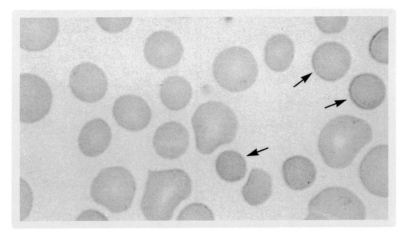

Fig. 8.13 Hereditary spherocytosis. Spherocytes are smaller and thicker than normal red cells but only totally spherical in extreme cases (courtesy Professor Victor Hoffbrand and Dr John Pettit).

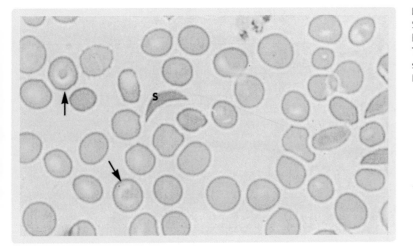

Fig. 8.14 Sickle-cell anaemia. Sickled cells are variable in shape, but classically are crescentic (**s**). Target cells are also commonly seen (courtesy Professor Victor Hoffbrand and Dr John Pettit).

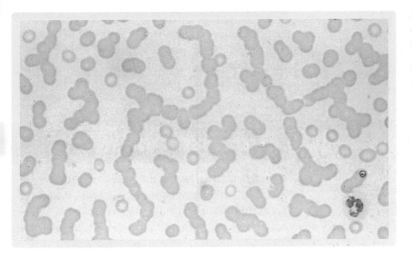

Fig. 8.15 Multiple myeloma. Red cell rouleaux (stacked cells) are seen due to the excess high-molecular-weight proteins in the blood (courtesy Professor Victor Hoffbrand and Dr John Pettit).

Fig. 8.16 Right shift. Using a neutrophil with a three-lobed nucleus as a marker for normal granulocyte maturation, a shift of development to either the right or left can be seen. Hypermature neutrophils (right shift) are seen in non-infectious inflammatory processes, e.g. malignancy, megaloblastic anaemia, iron deficiency, liver disease, uraemia. Left shift is indicated by the presence of immature 'band' forms which occur due to neutrophil leucocytosis. In this example left shift is due to abdominal sepsis (courtesy Professor Victor Hoffbrand and Dr John Pettit).

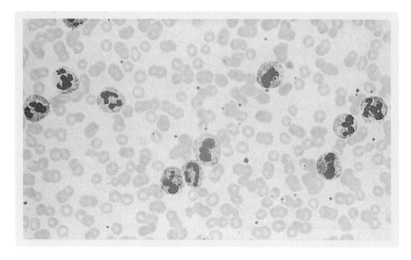

Fig. 8.17 Haemoglobin electrophoresis is used to detect different forms of haemoglobin (Hb). It can detect HbS (sickle haemoglobin), HbC, HbF (fetal haemoglobin), HbA (adult haemoglobin) and HbH (β tetramer, sometimes represented as β_4).

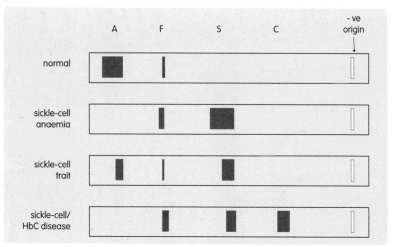

macrophages and erythroblasts. Fig. 8.18 shows a normal bone marrow smear.

Collection of bone marrow

- Aspiration of bone marrow involves the insertion of a hollow needle into the iliac crest or more rarely the sternum. Individual cell detail can be assessed from aspirates
- Trephine biopsy involves insertion of a large-bore needle into the iliac crest. A core of bone and marrow is obtained, which is examined as a histological specimen. These specimens are useful for assessing marrow architecture and cellularity.

The bone marrow findings in some disorders are listed in Fig. 8.19.

LYMPH NODE BIOPSY

Lymph nodes are biopsied for histological examination when malignancy is suspected. A lymph node biopsy from a patient with Hodgkin's lymphoma is shown in Fig. 8.20.

CYTOGENETIC ANALYSIS

Cytogenetic analysis is the study of structure and function of chromosomes. Certain cytogenetic abnormalities are strongly associated with specific conditions. Important examples in haematology are:

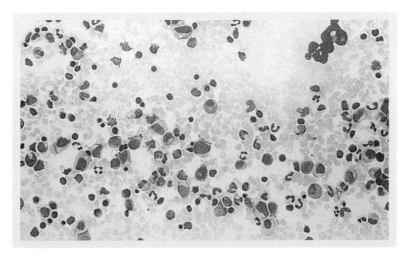

Fig. 8.18 Normal bone marrow smear. Haemopoietic cells and supporting reticuloendothelial cells are usually seen (courtesy Professor Victor Hoffbrand and Dr John Pettit).

Fig. 8.19 Appearance of the bone marrow in some haematological disorders

Disorder	Bone marrow appearance
Iron-deficiency anaemia	Absent iron stores from macrophages
Megaloblastic anaemia	Hypercellular marrow with megaloblasts present; giant metamyelocytes often seen
Haemolytic anaemia	Hypercellular marrow with erythroid hyperplasia; reduced myeloid/erythroid ratio (usually 2–8)
Aplastic anaemia	Hypocellular marrow
Acute leukaemia	Hypercellular marrow infiltrated with blasts
Chronic lymphocytic leukaemia	Hypercellular marrow with lymphocytic infiltration
Chronic myeloid leukaemia	Hypercellular marrow with granulocytic and megakaryocytic hyperplasia
Multiple myeloma	Increased proportion of plasma cells (often abnormal)
Polycythaemia rubra vera and essential thrombocythaemia	Hypercellular marrow with hyperplasia of all cell lineages
Myelofibrosis	Early—hypercellularity, late—reactive fibrosis of the bone marrow and reduced haemopoiesis

Courtesy Professor Victor Hoffbrand and Dr John Pettit.

- t(9;22): this is found in chronic myeloid leukaemia (the altered chromosome 22 is called the Philadelphia chromosome)
- t(14;18): this is associated with follicle centre lymphomas
- t(8;14): this is associated with Burkitt's lymphoma.

ESR AND PLASMA VISCOSITY

The erythrocyte sedimentation rate (ESR) is the rate of fall of a column of red cells in plasma over 1 hour. The normal range in men is 1–5 mm/hour and in women it is 5–15 mm/hour. ESR is raised with increased plasma viscosity, which is a more easily automated test. The concentration of proteins (fibrinogen and globulins) in the plasma is the major determinant of viscosity. ESR and plasma viscosity are used as indicators of the acute phase response. ESR is raised in inflammation (including response to infection), malignancy (including myeloma) and anaemia. It is important to remember that a normal increase in ESR occurs with age and during pregnancy.

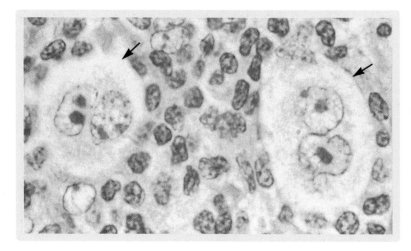

Fig. 8.20 Hodgkin's lymphoma on lymph node biopsy showing two binucleate Reed–Sternberg cells (arrows). Demonstration of Reed–Sternberg cells (or variants) against a background of inflammatory cells is required to diagnose Hodgkin's lymphoma (courtesy Professor Victor Hoffbrand and Dr John Pettit).

Fig. 8.21 Tests of the coagulation cascade

Text	Normal range	Causes of abnormalities
Thrombin time	10–12 seconds	Heparin therapy DIC Afibrinogenaemia
Prothrombin time	12–14 seconds	Deficiencies of factor VII Liver disease Warfarin therapy DIC
Activated partial thromboplastin time	30–40 seconds	Deficiencies of factors VIII, IX, XI, XII von Willebrand's disease DIC Heparin therapy
PT and APTT	Prolonged	Deficiencies of factors II, V, X

DIC, disseminated intravascular coagulation.

SERUM ELECTROPHORESIS

Normal serum proteins

Proteins in the plasma are vital to maintain colloid osmotic pressure and circulating volume (albumin), to respond to infectious challenges (globulins), for haemostasis (clotting factors) and for transport (e.g. transferrin). These proteins can be distinguished by electrophoresis to produce several bands, including:

- Albumin
- α_1-antitrypsin
- α_2-macroglobulin, haptoglobin
- β-transferrin
- γ-globulins.

Acute phase proteins

Following a variety of insults, the liver synthesizes increased quantities of proteins. These proteins, normally present in serum in small amounts, include:

- α_1-antitrypsin
- Fibrinogen
- Complement
- Haptoglobin
- C-reactive protein.

ESR and plasma viscosity indirectly measure the acute phase response by detecting changes in the 'thickness' of plasma. C-reactive protein (CRP) can be measured directly. CRP changes more rapidly than ESR (it will fall within 2–3 days of recovery), so is more sensitive to changes in the response to therapy or in disease activity. Unlike ESR, CRP is not raised in pregnancy or anaemia.

CLOTTING TESTS

Prothrombin time (PT), activated partial thromboplastin time (APPT) and thrombin time are tests of the function of the coagulation cascade. A summary of their normal range and the causes of abnormal results are shown in Fig. 8.21.

Specific factor assays can be used to identify deficiencies of single coagulation factors. This is of relevance to haemophilia when an assay can indicate the level of factor in the blood and therefore severity of disease.

Fibrinogen degradation products are used to identify clots, e.g. post-DVT/disseminated intravascular coagulation. Most laboratories nowadays report these as D-dimers which is one way of measuring FDPs. These clotting tests are discussed in Chapter 6.

Prolonged APPT with a normal PT is found in:
- Lupus anticoagulant
- Deficiencies of factors VIII, IX, XI and XII.

Prolonged PT with a normal APPT is found in:
- Factor VI deficiency
- Liver disease
- Warfarin (at therapeutic dose).

SELF-ASSESSMENT

Indicate whether each answer is true or false.

1. **Which of the following characteristics of tumour cells can activate an immune response:**
   a. Viral antigens.
   b. Embryonic antigens.
   c. Glycosylated variants of normal self-proteins.
   d. Absence of MHC class I molecules.
   e. High concentrations of normal self-proteins.

2. **Regarding the immune system:**
   a. An antigen is a molecule that can be recognized by the adaptive immune system.
   b. Antibody isotypes are antibodies that bind to other antibodies.
   c. Haptens are not immunogenic by themselves.
   d. Lymph nodes are primary lymphoid organs.
   e. The innate immune system exhibits immunological memory.

3. **In comparison to monocytes, macrophages:**
   a. Are smaller.
   b. Live longer.
   c. Have greater phagocytic ability.
   d. Are more likely to be found in the circulation.
   e. Produce more lytic enzymes.

4. **Macrophages can be activated by:**
   a. Interferon-γ.
   b. Complement.
   c. Coagulation products.
   d. Interleukin-2.
   e. Fas ligand.

5. **In comparison to macrophages, neutrophils:**
   a. Are longer lived.
   b. Can control mycobacteria.
   c. Communicate with T cells.
   d. Can present exogenous antigen.
   e. Move and phagocytose more quickly.

6. **Which of the following are products of oxygen-dependent pathways:**
   a. Superoxide radicals.
   b. Hypochlorous acid.
   c. Lysozyme.
   d. Hydrogen peroxide.
   e. Cationic proteins.

7. **Concerning natural killer cells:**
   a. They are activated by specific, individual antigens.
   b. They can detect classical and non-classical MHC class I molecules.
   c. They are involved in antibody-dependent cell-mediated cytotoxicity.
   d. Because they are lymphoid cells, they exhibit immunological memory.
   e. They cause cellular necrosis.

8. **Concerning the complement system:**
   a. The classical pathway is activated by MHC molecules.
   b. It can be activated by bacterial carbohydrates.
   c. It can activate spontaneously.
   d. It causes ion-permeable pores to form in target cells.
   e. It is involved in the recruitment of inflammatory cells.

9. **Which of the following inhibitors of complement are linked with the correct actions:**
   a. Factor H inactivates C5 convertase.
   b. Decay accelerating factor speeds up the decay of the membrane attack complex.
   c. Factor I cleaves C3b and C4b.
   d. CD59 prevents the membrane attack complex from forming.
   e. C1 inhibitor inhibits C1.

10. **Which of the following are members of the immunoglobulin gene superfamily:**
    a. T cell receptor.
    b. CD3-ζ.
    c. Human leucocyte antigen molecules.
    d. ICAM-1.
    e. Polyimmunoglobulin receptor.

11. **Concerning primary and secondary lymphoid tissue:**
    a. The thymus is a secondary lymphoid organ.
    b. Lymph node germinal follicles contain mainly T cells.
    c. B-cell hypermutation occurs in the bone marrow.
    d. Lymph nodes sample antigen from the blood.
    e. Peyer's patches are part of the mucosal-associated lymphoid tissue.

12. Concerning generation of antigen receptor diversity:

   a. Both the light and heavy immunoglobulin chain variable regions are encoded by V, D and J gene segments.
   b. Diversity can only be generated before encountering antigen.
   c. Somatic hypermutation occurs in both B and T cells.
   d. Antibodies produced late in an immune response have increased affinity for antigen.
   e. Each person's T cell receptor repertoire will be the same.

13. IgA:

   a. Is important in mucosal immunity.
   b. Is found in breast milk.
   c. Is the most abundant immunoglobulin in the blood.
   d. Crosses the placenta.
   e. Is normally a dimer.

14. The major histocompatibility complex (MHC):

   a. Encodes human leucocyte antigen (HLA) molecules.
   b. Is located on chromosome 16 in humans.
   c. Encodes some complement components.
   d. Contains the gene for TNF.
   e. Encodes β_2-microglobulin.

15. Concerning the acute phase response:

   a. There is a change in the concentration of a number of plasma proteins.
   b. Leucocytosis and thrombocytopenia develop.
   c. Levels of caeruloplasmin and α_1-glycoprotein undergo a 100–1000-fold increase.
   d. Levels of C-reactive protein and serum amyloid A (SAA) rise within hours of tissue injury.
   e. There is a decrease in plasma viscosity.

16. Concerning class I MHC molecules:

   a. A class I molecule is made up of α- and β-chains.
   b. CD8$^+$ T cells are class I MHC-restricted.
   c. Class I molecules are present only on antigen-presenting cells.
   d. Class I molecules present endogenous antigen.
   e. A class I molecule can bind longer peptides than a class II molecule because the peptide-binding cleft is more open.

17. Concerning recognition molecules of the immune system:

   a. Immunoglobulin molecules consist of two heavy chains and two light chains.
   b. The variable regions of the heavy and light chains are identical.
   c. The framework regions of immunoglobulins comprise the antigen-binding site.
   d. TCR signals are transduced by $Ig\alpha/Ig\beta$.
   e. Approximately 95% of T cells express $\gamma\delta$ receptors.

18. The following are components of the innate immune system:

   a. Interferons α and β.
   b. T cells.
   c. Complement.
   d. Antibody.
   e. Acute phase proteins.

19. DiGeorge syndrome is characterized by:

   a. Malformation of the third and fourth pharyngeal pouches.
   b. Thymic hyperplasia.
   c. Hyperparathyroidism.
   d. Cardiac defects.
   e. Recurrent infections.

20. Regarding the complement system:

   a. Complement components are proteins or glycoproteins.
   b. Complement can only be activated by the alternative and classical pathways.
   c. The alternative pathway is usually activated by IgM and IgG.
   d. Complement components C5, C6, C7, C8 and C9 comprise the membrane attack complex.
   e. The conversion of C3 to C3b by C3 convertase is the major amplification process in the complement cascade.

21. Concerning lymph nodes:

   a. Antigen enters lymph nodes from the blood.
   b. Lymph filters from the cortex to the medulla.
   c. They contain B cells, T cells and antigen-presenting cells.
   d. Lymphocytes can enter the node directly from the blood.
   e. They act to pump lymph around the body.

22. The following are examples of mucosal-associated lymphoid tissue (MALT):

   a. Tonsils.
   b. Appendix.
   c. Thymus.
   d. Peyer's patches.
   e. Inguinal lymph nodes.

23. The thymus:

   a. Is a bilobed gland.
   b. Is usually located in the neck.
   c. Exhibits a high rate of cell death.
   d. Contains stromal cells that support developing neutrophils.
   e. Produces hormones that control T cell maturation.

24. **T helper cells:**
    a. Express CD4.
    b. Are required for antibody production against protein antigens.
    c. Produce a wide variety of cytokines, which stimulate the innate and adaptive immune systems.
    d. Do not express T cell receptors.
    e. Determine the type of adaptive immune response mounted.

25. **Concerning acute inflammation:**
    a. Acute inflammation is characterized by infiltration of neutrophils and vascular changes.
    b. TNF-α is an important mediator.
    c. The complement system does not play a role.
    d. The coagulation and fibrinolytic systems are activated.
    e. ICAM-1 and ICAM-2 are downregulated.

26. **The actions of cytokines in acute inflammation include:**
    a. Induction of adhesion molecules.
    b. Induction of cell membrane phospholipid and prostaglandin metabolism.
    c. Chemotaxis of neutrophils.
    d. Stimulate fibroblast proliferation.
    e. Mediate the acute phase response.

27. **Which of the following are arachidonic acid metabolites:**
    a. Platelet-activating factor.
    b. Leukotriene B$_4$.
    c. Thromboxane A$_2$.
    d. Perforin.
    e. Prostacyclin.

28. **Concerning leucocyte margination and extravasation in acute inflammation:**
    a. Neutrophils are important in the early part of the response.
    b. Selectin molecules expressed constitutively on endothelial cells bind to selectin molecules on leucocytes.
    c. The interaction between leucocytes and endothelium is strengthened by integrin molecules.
    d. Integrin molecules are important for leucocyte homing.
    e. The endothelial cells form pores large enough for spherical leucocytes to pass through.

29. **Concerning chronic inflammation:**
    a. Neutrophils form the majority of cells present.
    b. The macrophage plays a central role.
    c. Granuloma formation is a characteristic feature.
    d. TNF-α is crucial in granuloma maintenance.
    e. Lymphocytes are not usually present.

30. **The following are potential consequences of chronic inflammation:**
    a. Tissue injury.
    b. The tissue returns to normal.
    c. Weight loss and fever.
    d. Adaptive immune system activation.
    e. Fibrosis.

31. **Which of the following are important for the immune response to viruses:**
    a. Lysozyme.
    b. Antibody.
    c. Interferons.
    d. Eosinophils.
    e. Cytotoxic T cells.

32. **Viruses evade the normal immune response by:**
    a. Undergoing mutation between epidemics.
    b. Reducing MHC class I expression.
    c. Mutating within the host.
    d. Releasing exotoxins.
    e. Becoming latent.

33. **Protozoal infection is often chronic because:**
    a. They have marked antigenic variation.
    b. They are immunosuppressive.
    c. They have complex lifecycles.
    d. Infection is intracellular.
    e. They can escape into the cytoplasm following phagocytosis.

34. **Regarding hypersensitivity reactions:**
    a. Type I hypersensitivity reactions are mediated by IgG.
    b. Type III hypersensitivity involves the formation of immune complexes.
    c. Mast cells play a key role in immediate hypersensitivity.
    d. Delayed-type hypersensitivity mechanisms play a key role in haemolytic disease of the newborn due to rhesus incompatibility.
    e. The Arthus reaction is a localized type III reaction.

35. **The following are examples of hypersensitivity reactions:**
    a. A positive skin-prick test.
    b. A positive Mantoux or Heaf test.
    c. Hay fever.
    d. Graves' disease.
    e. Osteoarthritis.

36. **Concerning anti-inflammatory drugs:**
    a. Paracetamol is an excellent anti-inflammatory.
    b. Steroids can only be given intravenously.
    c. NSAIDs act by inhibiting phospholipase A$_2$.
    d. Anti-TNF-α is anti-inflammatory.
    e. NSAIDs may be nephrotoxic and cause bronchospasm.

37. Concerning allergies:

a. They are always type I hypersensitivity reactions.
b. Asthma is characterized by reversible airway obstruction.
c. Pollen and dust-mite faeces are common allergens.
d. Atopy refers to a predisposition to allergic conditions.
e. Anaphylaxis is associated with hypertension.

38. Concerning treatment of allergies:

a. Controlled exposure to low doses of antigen can be helpful.
b. Antihistamines cure many allergic conditions.
c. Steroids are useful.
d. Adrenaline is commonly needed in the treatment of severe anaphylaxis.
e. Prophylactic treatment often reduces the occurrence of symptoms.

39. Self-tolerance can be due to:

a. Early clonal deletion.
b. Clonal anergy.
c. Molecular mimicry.
d. Fas ligand expression.
e. Regulatory T cells.

40. Concerning systemic lupus erythematous (SLE):

a. SLE is an organ-specific autoimmune disease.
b. SLE is more common in men than in women.
c. SLE is characterized by antinuclear autoantibodies.
d. The presence of HLA-DR5 and HLA-DR6 haplotypes confers an increased risk of developing SLE.
e. An erythematous rash is common.

41. Concerning rheumatoid arthritis (RA):

a. RA is characterized by inflammation of the synovium and destruction of the articular cartilage.
b. Inflammation is limited to joints.
c. TNF is a key cytokine in pathogenesis.
d. RA is more common in women than in men.
e. Type II collagen is the major autoantigen.

42. Rheumatoid factor:

a. Is found in all cases of rheumatoid arthritis.
b. Is an autoantibody.
c. Is directed against IgM.
d. Can activate complement.
e. Amplifies the inflammatory response.

43. The following autoimmune diseases are organ specific:

a. Reiter's syndrome.
b. Hashimoto's thyroiditis.
c. Myasthenia gravis.
d. Graves' disease.
e. Polyarteritis nodosa.

44. The following are examples of primary immunodeficiencies:

a. Chronic granulomatous disease.
b. Transient hypogammaglobulinaemia of infancy.
c. Splenectomy.
d. AIDS.
e. Wiskott–Aldrich syndrome.

45. Antibody deficiency can present with:

a. Bronchiectasis.
b. Diarrhoea.
c. Rheumatoid arthritis.
d. Hyperviscosity.
e. *Mycoplasma* joint infections.

46. Features of HIV include:

a. Polyclonal B cell activation.
b. Defective T cell function.
c. Low rate of viral replication during asymptomatic phase.
d. Antibodies directed against gp120 and gp41.
e. Persistent generalized lymphadenopathy.

47. During HIV infection, which of the following infections are common:

a. CMV retinitis.
b. *Pneumocystis carinii*.
c. Oesophageal candidiasis.
d. *Mycobacterium avium intracellulare* (MAC).
e. Toxoplasmosis.

48. Concerning the routine immunization schedule in the UK:

a. MMR is given at 2, 3 and 4 months.
b. BCG is given neonatally or at 10–14 years.
c. Influenza vaccine is given to people over 65 years of age.
d. Meningococcal vaccine is given before the child goes to school.
e. Tetanus vaccine requires boosters.

49. Live vaccines are used to prevent:

a. Polio.
b. Tetanus.
c. Tuberculosis.
d. Rubella.
e. Hepatitis B.

50. Concerning mechanisms of transplant rejection:

a. Hyperacute rejection only occurs once the recipient has synthesized antibody to the graft.
b. Acute cellular rejection is primarily mediated by natural killer cells.
c. Acute rejection is due to anti-donor antibodies.
d. Chronic rejection may be due to several mechanisms.
e. Complement is implicated in hyperacute rejection.

51. **The risk of transplant rejection can be reduced by:**

    a. Using a graft from a monozygous twin.
    b. Using steroids.
    c. Using monoclonal antibodies.
    d. Prompt cooling of transplanted organs.
    e. Using unmatched grafts.

52. **Bone marrow:**

    a. Is the main site of haemopoiesis in adults.
    b. Is found throughout the skeleton of newborns.
    c. Contains a large amount of fat.
    d. Contains macrophages important for the transfer of iron to developing erythrocytes.
    e. Forms T lymphocyte precursors.

53. **Regarding the spleen:**

    a. The spleen is normally anterior to the stomach.
    b. The red pulp removes old or defective erythrocytes from the circulation.
    c. There are usually more primary than secondary B cell follicles.
    d. The spleen develops from the primitive gut.
    e. Primary cancers are rare.

54. **Haemopoietic stem cells:**

    a. Are found only in the bone marrow.
    b. Are able to produce plasma cells.
    c. Can self-replicate.
    d. Become lineage-committed precursor cells.
    e. Need growth factors to differentiate.

55. **Concerning disorders of the spleen:**

    a. Congestive splenomegaly is caused by persistent venous congestion.
    b. Splenomegaly in the UK is usually due to parasitic infection.
    c. Splenic infarction occurs in myeloproliferative disorders.
    d. Epstein–Barr virus infection is linked to splenic rupture.
    e. The spleen may be affected by haematological neoplasms.

56. **Splenectomy is indicated in:**

    a. Splenic rupture.
    b. Splenic tumours.
    c. Idiopathic thrombocytopenic purpura.
    d. Autoimmune haemolytic anaemia.
    e. Splenic cysts.

57. **Hereditary spherocytosis is characterized by:**

    a. An autosomal dominant pattern of inheritance.
    b. Intravascular haemolysis.
    c. The presence of spherocytes on the peripheral blood film smear.
    d. Increased osmotic fragility of red cells.
    e. Decreased autohaemolysis of red cells.

58. **Features of β-thalassaemia major include:**

    a. A microcytic, hypochromic anaemia.
    b. High serum iron.
    c. Increased red-cell lifespan.
    d. Homozygosity for defective genes causing reduced β-chain production.
    e. HbA on electrophoresis.

59. **Erythrocytes:**

    a. Have a bilobed nucleus.
    b. Are derived from the CFU-GEMM precursor.
    c. Transport CO_2.
    d. Have an average lifespan of 50 days.
    e. Are usually spherical.

60. **Concerning iron metabolism:**

    a. Iron is absorbed in the stomach.
    b. Excess iron is readily excreted.
    c. Iron is transported in the blood bound to apoferritin.
    d. Primary haemochromatosis is caused by excessive intestinal absorption.
    e. Total body stores of iron are 4 kg.

61. **Concerning haemoglobin:**

    a. Adult haemoglobin is composed of four identical polypeptide subunits.
    b. Oxygen is transported bound to haem.
    c. The Bohr effect (a shift of the oxygen dissociation curve) is due to increased H^+.
    d. Oxygen binding follows a sigmoidal curve.
    e. 2,3-diphosphoglycerate levels rise in hypoxia to allow increased oxygen uptake by haemoglobin.

62. **Vitamin B_{12}:**

    a. Is absorbed in the proximal jejunum.
    b. Contains cobalt.
    c. Absorption is reduced following total gastrectomy.
    d. Requires extrinsic factor for absorption.
    e. Is synthesized by the skin.

63. **Regarding folic acid:**

    a. It is found in vegetables.
    b. It is absorbed in the colon.
    c. 50 mg per day is the normal daily requirement.
    d. Deficiency may occur in coeliac disease.
    e. The requirement decreases during pregnancy.

64. **A normochromic normocytic anaemia is commonly associated with:**

    a. Iron deficiency.
    b. Tuberculosis.
    c. Rheumatoid arthritis.
    d. Vitamin B_{12} deficiency.
    e. Thalassaemia.

65. Which of the following are features of iron-deficiency anaemia?

a. Glossitis.
b. Koilonychia.
c. Macrocytic, hypochromic anaemia.
d. Reduced serum ferritin.
e. Reduced serum transferrin.

66. Causes of absolute polycythaemia include:

a. Polycythaemia rubra vera.
b. Dehydration.
c. Renal carcinoma.
d. Cyanotic heart disease.
e. Diuretic therapy.

67. Which of the following are red-cell precursors:

a. Pronormoblast.
b. Normoblast.
c. Stomatocyte.
d. Reticulocyte.
e. Echinocyte.

68. Which of the following are features of haemolytic anaemias:

a. Pigment gallstones.
b. Raised serum haptoglobin.
c. Haemosiderinuria.
d. Haemoglobinaemia.
e. Reticulocytosis.

69. Which of the following can precipitate haemolysis in glucose-6-phosphate dehydrogenase deficiency?

a. Infection.
b. Alkalosis.
c. Primaquine.
d. Fava beans.
e. Normal saline.

70. Management of sickle-cell anaemia can include:

a. Vaccinations.
b. Folic acid.
c. Antibiotics.
d. Blood transfusions.
e. Fluids.

71. Fetal haemoglobin:

a. Has a sigmoidal oxygen dissociation curve.
b. Has a lower affinity for oxygen than adult haemoglobin.
c. May be raised in β-thalassaemia syndromes.
d. Is produced by the fetal liver.
e. Is composed of two α- and two β-chains.

72. Erythropoietin:

a. Prevents apoptosis of developing erythrocyte precursors.
b. Is produced in the bone marrow.
c. Is raised in chronic hypoxia.
d. May be used iatrogenically.
e. Is needed for white cell maturation.

73. Aplastic anaemia can be:

a. Iatrogenic.
b. Part of a congenital syndrome.
c. Associated with acute infection.
d. Associated with increased bone marrow cellularity.
e. Treated with testosterone.

74. In haemolytic anaemia:

a. Red-cell fragmentation can be associated with prosthetic heart valves.
b. Acute renal failure can occur.
c. Urinary bilirubin is increased.
d. Urinary urobilinogen is increased.
e. A microcytosis is common.

75. Polymorphonuclear leucocytes:

a. Have a large round nucleus.
b. Primarily respond to parasitic infections.
c. Are granulocytes.
d. Are phagocytic.
e. Are a major constituent of pus.

76. Myelodysplastic syndromes:

a. Are acquired neoplastic disorders of the bone marrow.
b. Are due to defects in fully differentiated cells.
c. May progress to acute myeloid leukaemia.
d. Are commonest in children.
e. Have a worse prognosis when blasts account for more than 5% of the bone marrow.

77. Leucostatic symptoms:

a. Occur in leukaemia.
b. Are caused by fat embolism.
c. Include retinal haemorrhage.
d. Include a reduced level of consciousness.
e. Resolve if the white-cell count increases.

78. Which of the following are consistent with a diagnosis of non-Hodgkin's lymphoma:

a. Painless lymphadenopathy.
b. Reed–Sternberg cells in the lesion.
c. Fever, night sweats and weight loss.
d. Fanconi's syndrome.
e. HIV infection.

79. Which of the following are myeloproliferative conditions:

a. Polycythaemia rubra vera.
b. Sideroblastic anaemia.
c. Myelofibrosis.
d. Primary thrombocythaemia.
e. Acute lymphoblastic leukaemia.

80. A macrophage:

a. Is a differentiated monocyte.
b. Is capable of phagocytosis.
c. May play an important role in the adaptive immune response.
d. Can be infected by HIV.
e. Is central to the allergic response.

81. **Chronic lymphocytic leukaemia:**
    a. Is the most common leukaemia.
    b. Is rapidly progressive.
    c. Is usually B cell in origin.
    d. Is commonly associated with autoimmune haemolytic anaemia.
    e. Converts to acute leukaemia within 5 years.

82. **Regarding acute lymphoblastic leukaemia:**
    a. It is the most common leukaemia in children.
    b. Presentation after 10 years of age is associated with a poorer prognosis.
    c. Remission rates are low.
    d. It is commonly T cell in origin.
    e. It may be caused by radiation exposure.

83. **Acute myeloblastic leukaemia:**
    a. Is caused by an accumulation of differentiated myeloid cells in the bone marrow.
    b. Is associated with Down syndrome.
    c. Is characterized by isochromosome 12p.
    d. Has a better prognosis in older patients.
    e. May present with bleeding.

84. **Regarding chronic myeloid leukaemia:**
    a. It is often identified in chronic phase.
    b. Less than 10% of patients develop to an accelerated phase within 10 years of diagnosis.
    c. The Philadelphia chromosome is a disease marker.
    d. Treatment may be with Glivec.
    e. Bone marrow transplant is potentially curative.

85. **Which of the following are features of multiple myeloma:**
    a. Bence Jones protein in the plasma.
    b. Presentation with paraplegia.
    c. Repeated infections.
    d. Bone destruction.
    e. >10% plasma cells in the marrow.

86. **Which of the following may cause a neutropenia:**
    a. Aplastic anaemia.
    b. Leukaemia.
    c. Kostmann's syndrome.
    d. Chemotherapy.
    e. Antimalarial drugs.

87. **Platelets:**
    a. Are derived from the nucleus of megakaryocytes.
    b. Are transported in the blood by von Willebrand's factor.
    c. Are involved in primary haemostasis.
    d. Can bind directly to collagen.
    e. Are inhibited by thromboxane A_2.

88. **Bleeding can occur as a consequence of:**
    a. Drug therapy.
    b. Chemotherapy and radiotherapy.
    c. X-linked diseases.
    d. Splenomegaly.
    e. Defective platelet adhesion.

89. **Concerning vitamin-K-dependent clotting factors:**
    a. Prothrombin is a vitamin-K-dependent clotting factor.
    b. Factor IX is vitamin K dependent.
    c. Vitamin K is required for post-translational acetylation.
    d. Vitamin K deficiency can be caused by fat malabsorption.
    e. Haemophilia A can be caused by vitamin K deficiency.

90. **Which of the following will cause the prothrombin time to be increased:**
    a. Disseminated intravascular coagulation.
    b. von Willebrand's disease.
    c. Vitamin K deficiency.
    d. Haemophilia A.
    e. Haemophilia B.

91. **Which of the following are associated with an increased risk of clotting:**
    a. Factor V Leiden.
    b. Disseminated cancer.
    c. Oestrogen therapy.
    d. Protein C deficiency.
    e. Prolonged immobilization.

92. **Idiopathic thrombocytopenic purpura:**
    a. Is characterized by IgA-positive petechiae.
    b. Is associated with anti-platelet antibodies in the plasma.
    c. Is associated with HIV disease.
    d. May be treated with high-dose glucocorticoids.
    e. May be treated with fresh-frozen plasma only.

93. **Heparin:**
    a. Is routinely given orally.
    b. Is routinely monitored using the international normalized ratio.
    c. Is a glycosaminoglycan.
    d. Has a different activity at different molecular weights.
    e. Is structurally related to warfarin.

94. **Which of the following limit thrombus formation:**
    a. Proteins C and S.
    b. Plasminogen activator inhibitor.
    c. Thrombocytopenia.
    d. Streptokinase.
    e. Christmas factor.

95. Regarding haemophilia A:

a. Inheritance is autosomal dominant.
b. Prevalence depends on social class.
c. It may be treated prophylactically with factor VII.
d. It is associated with pathological arthrodesis.
e. It may be mimicked by von Willebrand's disease.

96. Which of the following test results are in the normal range for peripheral venous blood in a healthy 25-year-old man:

a. Haemoglobin: 14 g/dL.
b. White-cell count: 8×10^9/L.
c. pO_2: 40 mmHg.
d. Reticulocyte count: 5% of peripheral red blood cells.
e. Platelets: 100×10^9/L.

97. Which of the following are detected on peripheral blood smears:

a. Howell–Jolly bodies.
b. Auer rods.
c. Philadelphia chromosome.
d. Reticulocytosis.
e. Bence Jones protein.

98. Regarding the ABO antigen system:

a. People who are blood group O must have two parents who are both blood group O.
b. People who are blood group A will produce anti-B antibodies.
c. In group O, the T antigen is left unchanged.
d. Group AB people will usually produce a haemolytic reaction to group O blood.
e. Anti-A and anti-B antibodies are usually IgG.

99. Haemolytic disease of the newborn:

a. Is commonly due to rhesus D incompatibility.
b. Usually occurs in the first child.
c. Will not occur if the mother is rhesus D positive.
d. Can be prevented by passive immunization.
e. Is due to IgM antibodies.

100. Regarding acute haemolytic transfusion reactions:

a. They are caused by the destruction of donor red blood cells by antibodies present in the recipient's serum.
b. They may lead to complement activation.
c. They develop a few days after transfusion.
d. Hypertension, flushing, urticaria, diarrhoea and vomiting ensue.
e. They may cause disseminated intravascular coagulation.

1. What are the differences between Th1 and Th2 cells?

2. Explain what the term 'positive and negative selection of T cells' means and state where these processes take place.

3. List the clinical features of haemolytic anaemias and explain how they arise.

4. Draw the structure of an immunoglobulin molecule and list the functions of immunoglobulins.

5. Write short notes on pernicious anaemia.

6. What is haemolytic disease of the newborn and how can it be prevented?

7. Define the following terms: innate and adaptive immunity; antigen; immunogen; hapten; epitope.

8. What are the differences between active and passive immunization? Outline the advantages and disadvantages of each.

9. Write short notes on the role of vitamin K in coagulation.

10. Draw and label a diagram of a platelet.

11. A 24-year-old intravenous drug user presents to casualty with weight loss, fever and 2 months of unproductive cough. A chest radiograph reveals bilateral hilar lymphadenopathy. A full blood count shows a haemoglobin of 8 g/dL with a normal neutrophil count and a total lymphocyte count of 0.1.

    a. What is the most likely diagnosis?
    b. How else may a patient with this condition have presented?
    c. What medications are available to treat his underlying condition?

12. A 65-year-old man presents with diffuse symmetrical lymphadenopathy and splenomegaly. He complains only of tiredness. A full blood count reveals a haemoglobin of 9 g/dL (normochromic, normocytic), and his total leucocyte count is 125 × 10^9/L, composed mostly of lymphocytes.

    a. What is the most likely diagnosis?
    b. How would you establish this diagnosis?
    c. How would you treat him, and what is his prognosis?

13. A 57-year-old man with lumbar back pain of 2 weeks' duration is brought into casualty, paraplegic after a minor fall. X-ray shows osteolytic lesions with vertebral collapse, and protein electrophoresis shows a paraprotein in his serum.

    a. What is the most likely diagnosis?
    b. What other clinical features might you expect this patient to exhibit?

14. A 15-year-old male presents with chronic sputum production and is found to have thickened bronchial walls on chest CT. The appearances are consistent with bronchiectasis. He also complains of recurrent gastrointestinal infections. His uncle died from bronchiectasis at the age of 35.

    a. What is the likely diagnosis?
    b. What treatment would you offer him?

15. You are involved in the care of a 20-year-old man who was involved in a motorbike accident and rushed to casualty by ambulance. Amongst his injuries he had fractured his 10th rib on the left hand side. The fractured bone had ruptured his spleen and it was necessary to perform an emergency splenectomy. What advice would you give him about his prognosis?

16. A 63-year-old Caucasian woman presents with a severe pyrexia of unknown origin. She has irregular peaks of fever and profound malaise. Investigations reveal a CRP of 300 mg/L (normal 10 mg/L), haemoglobin 9 g/dL (normochromic, normocytic), albumin 14 g/L (normal 35–50 g/L) and polyclonal gammopathy. A chest CT taken 1 month previously revealed diffuse basal reticular shadowing, which, on repeat CT, progressed rapidly in parallel with the

patient's requirement for oxygen. All microbiological tests on broncho-alveolar lavage were negative and a transbronchial biopsy was negative. Bone marrow showed reactive changes only.

a. What test would you perform to establish the diagnosis?
b. What possible diagnoses might this test reveal?

---

17. An 18-year-old haemophiliac who has been well maintained haematologically in the UK went to Nepal following his A-levels. During this time he fell over and required treatment with blood products exceeding those he had taken with him. He presents with fever, maculopapular rash, splenomegaly and mouth ulcers 8 weeks after returning to the UK. He is severely lymphopenic with normal polymorphonuclear count and haemogloblin.

a. What blood products may he have received?
b. What prime diagnosis must be excluded?

---

18. A 20-year-old white Caucasian male who had dropped out of university was sent by his mother to a health food farm where he received a diet of broad beans. Two days after arriving he developed jaundice but initially had normal coloured urine, which changed to red after 1 day.

a. What is the likely diagnosis?
b. What would urine tests show?
c. What would be the salient changes in blood tests?

19. A 40-year-old man presents with a right hemiplegia. On examination he has a ruddy complexion and no movement in his right arm and leg. He has no previous history of serious disease. He is afebrile, has no cardiac murmurs and is not hypertensive.

a. What is the first urgent test you require and why?
b. Polycythaemia rubra vera is considered likely. What other investigations should you carry out?
c. If a diagnosis of polycythaemia rubra vera is confirmed, how would you manage this patient?

---

20. A 15-year-old bee-keeper's daughter presents to casualty 15 minutes after being stung by a bee. She has severely obstructed breathing caused by laryngeal oedema and is becoming cyanosed.

a. What is the most likely diagnosis?
b. How would you treat her?

For each scenario described below, choose the *single* most likely match from the list of options.
Each option may be used once, more than once, or not at all.

1. Concerning complement:

A. Alternative pathway
B. C3
C. Lectin pathway
D. Collectins
E. Anaphylotoxin
F. C1 esterase inhibitor
G. Membrane attack complex
H. C7
I. Classical pathway
J. Complement inhibitors

Instruction: For each scenario described below, choose the **single** most likely match from the above list of options. Each option may be used once, more than once, or not at all.

1. Final set of complement proteins, which form a polymer that punches holes in cell membranes. ☐

2. The initiation of complement proteins by antibodies. ☐

3. Deficient in hereditary angioedema. ☐

4. Causes increased vascular permeability and attracts white blood cells to the site of infection. ☐

5. Regulates the processes involved in the complement cascade. ☐

2. Concerning immunization:

A. Passive immunity
B. Plasma cells
C. Dead vaccine
D. Subunit vaccine
E. Innate immunity
F. Active immunity
G. Memory cells
H. Adjuvant
I. Pathogen
J. Live attenuated vaccine

Instruction: For each scenario described below, choose the **single** most likely match from the above list of options. Each option may be used once, more than once, or not at all.

1. A chemical that provides a danger signal to the innate immune system by causing low grade inflammation. ☐

2. Type of immunity targeted by vaccination. ☐

3. Cells which form from clonal expansion of B and T lymphocytes in vaccination, which are activated in a secondary immune response. ☐

4. The transfer of immunoglobulins to an individual. ☐

5. Form of vaccine that requires an adjuvant. ☐

3. Concerning cell surface molecules:

A. B cell receptor
B. Toll-like receptor
C. MHC class I
D. FAS ligand
E. T cell receptor
F. MHC class II
G. Antigen
H. Cell adhesion molecules (CAMs)
I. CD3
J. Collectins

Instruction: For each scenario described below, choose the **single** most likely match from the above list of options. Each option may be used once, more than once, or not at all.

1. Substances recognized by the specific receptors of the adaptive immune system. ☐

2. Pattern recognition molecules found in solution. ☐

3. Molecule to which peptide antigens from intracellular pathogens are directed. ☐

4. Molecule that recognizes intracellular or phagocytosed antigen when it is expressed simultaneously with the MHC in which it is lying. ☐

5. Family of related molecules found on mammalian cell surfaces which, upon recognizing a pathogen, activate the innate immune system. ☐

4. Concerning immunoglobulins:

A. IgA
B. J-chain
C. Type II hypersensitivity
D. IgM
E. Type I hypersensitivity
F. Type IV hypersensitivity
G. Class switch
H. IgG
I. Type III hypersensitivity
J. Clonal expansion

Instruction: For each scenario described below, choose the **single** most likely match from the above list of options. Each option may be used once, more than once, or not at all.

1. Process by which a single B cell can produce different classes of immunoglobulins. ☐

2. Antibody secreted onto mucosal surfaces. ☐

3. Immune response stimulated by the presence of allergens. ☐

4. Immunoglobulin from which all other immunoglobulins are derived in the process of class switch. ☐

5. Reaction of ABO antigens and antibodies in the blood. ☐

5. Concerning B and T lymphocytes:

A. CD8
B. Myeloid stem cells
C. Plasma cells
D. Basophil
E. Memory B cells
F. T helper cells
G. Cytotoxic T cells
H. Memory T cells
I. CD40
J. Lymphoid stem cells

Instruction: For each scenario described below, choose the **single** most likely match from the above list of options. Each option may be used once, more than once, or not at all.

1. Induces B cells to become fully active and begin releasing antibody. ☐

2. Cells from which B and T lymphocytes originate. ☐

3. Cells with a vast amount of endoplasmic reticulum in order to secrete large quantities of immunoglobulin. ☐

4. Cell marker associated with cytotoxic T cells. ☐

5. Cells which recognize antigen in conjunction with MHC class I. ☐

6. Concerning anaemia:

A. Iron
B. Folate deficiency anaemia
C. Erythrocyte
D. Folate
E. Pernicious anaemia
F. Aplastic anaemia
G. Vitamin B_{12}
H. Sickle cell anaemia
I. Sideroblastic anaemia
J. Iron-deficiency anaemia

Instruction: For each scenario described below, choose the **single** most likely match from the above list of options. Each option may be used once, more than once, or not at all.

1. Anaemia caused by a reduction in number and function of bone marrow stem cells. ☐

2. An anaemia which occurs frequently in women of reproductive age. ☐

3. The Schilling test is used to diagnose the cause of a deficiency of this substance. ☐

4. Anaemia presenting as chronic atrophic gastritis with a probable autoimmune aetiology. ☐

5. Inherited haemoglobinopathy causing elongation of the red cells into a rigid shape. ☐

7. Concerning haematological investigations:

A. Cytogenetic analysis
B. Prothrombin time (PT)
C. Fine needle aspiration
D. Differential white count
E. Erythrocyte sedimentation rate (ESR)
F. Full blood count
G. Serum electrophoresis
H. Bone marrow smear
I. Lymph node biopsy
J. Peripheral blood film

Instruction: For each scenario described below, choose the **single** most likely match from the above list of options. Each option may be used once, more than once, or not at all.

1. Test which allows the examination of different stages of haemopoiesis. ☐

2. The identification of specific levels of neutrophils, lymphocytes, monocytes, eosinophils and basophils in the blood. ☐

3. The rate of fall of a column of red blood cells in plasma over 1 hour. ☐

4. A test to measure the function of the coagulation cascade. ☐

5. The study of the structure and function of chromosomes to highlight any abnormalities which may indicate a certain condition. ☐

8. Concerning red blood cells:

A. Haemoglobin
B. Erythropoiesis
C. Bilirubin
D. Normoblasts
E. Erythropoietin (EPO)
F. Haemostasis
G. Transferrin
H. Erythrocyte
I. Reticulocyte
J. Haemopoietic stem cells

Instruction: For each scenario described below, choose the **single** most likely match from the above list of options. Each option may be used once, more than once, or not at all.

1. Highly glycosylated polypeptide hormone that stimulates the differentiation and maturation of erythrocytes. ☐

2. Red blood cell component comprising two α-chains with either two β- or two δ-chains. ☐

3. Breakdown product of red blood cells, which is conjugated in the liver and excreted in bile. ☐

4. Immature red blood cells, present in the bone marrow, and in low numbers in the bloodstream. ☐

5. Process by which red blood cells are made in the bone marrow. ☐

9. Concerning white blood cells:

A. Chronic myeloid leukaemia
B. Leucopenia
C. Monocytes
D. Neutrophils
E. Lymphocytes
F. Non-Hodgkin's lymphoma
G. Eosinophils
H. Hodgkin's disease
I. Mast cells
J. Basophils

Instruction: For each scenario described below, choose the **single** most likely match from the above list of options. Each option may be used once, more than once, or not at all.

1. Large, circulating white blood cells, with distinctive, kidney-shaped nuclei. ☐

2. A myeloproliferative disorder resulting from proliferation of multipotent myeloid stem cells. ☐

3. The first cells recruited to a site of acute inflammation. ☐

4. Cells which mediate the delayed stage in type I hypersensitivity. ☐

5. Condition characterized by the presence of pathognomonic Reed–Sternberg cells or derivatives, typically mixed with a variable inflammatory infiltrate. ☐

10. Concerning haemostasis:

A. Intrinsic pathway
B. Heparin
C. Platelets
D. Fibrin
E. Thrombocytopenia
F. Extrinsic pathway
G. Thrombin
H. Warfarin
I. Vitamin K
J. Anaemia

Instruction: For each scenario described below, choose the **single** most likely match from the above list of options. Each option may be used once, more than once, or not at all.

1. Substance that converts fibrinogen to fibrin in the final stages of the coagulation cascade. ☐

2. Vitamin K antagonist. ☐

3. Process of coagulation which occurs entirely within the circulation. ☐

4. A condition characterized by a decrease in the number of platelets in the blood. ☐

5. The stimulation of the coagulation cascade by tissue factor (TF), a glycoprotein present on fibroblasts. ☐

1. a. True Tumours induced by viral infection can express viral antigens.
   b. True Carcinoembryonic antigen is seen in colonic cancer, α-fetoprotein in liver cancers.
   c. True Normal cell proteins can become abnormally glycosylated in tumours.
   d. True Absence of MHC class I can stimulate NK cells.
   e. False Completely normal proteins cannot stimulate the immune system.

2. a. True Antigens are recognized by the adaptive immune system.
   b. False Isotypes are different classes of antibody.
   c. True Haptens require large carrier molecules to elicit an immune response.
   d. False Lymph nodes are secondary lymphoid organs.
   e. False The innate immune system does not exhibit memory.

3. a. False Macrophages are larger than monocytes.
   b. True Macrophages can survive for many years within the tissues.
   c. True Macrophages are primarily phagocytic.
   d. False Macrophages form from monocytes when they enter tissues.
   e. True Lytic enzymes are produced to improve destruction of phagocytosed material.

4. a. True Cytokines, including IFN-γ, activate macrophages.
   b. True Complement acts as an opsonin for phagocytes.
   c. True Coagulation products activate macrophages.
   d. False IL-2 is a T-cell growth factor.
   e. False Fas ligand will cause cells expressing Fas to undergo apoptosis.

5. a. False Macrophages are longer-lived; neutrophils die soon after dealing with pathogens.
   b. False Macrophages are required to control mycobacteria.
   c. False Macrophages, but not neutrophils, stimulate T cells by secreting IL-12.

d. False Neutrophils do not process exogenous antigen or produce MHC class II to present antigen.
e. True Neutrophils move and phagocytose more quickly than macrophages.

6. a. True Superoxide radicals are produced from molecular oxygen.
   b. True Hypochlorous acid is produced when myeloperoxidase catalyses a reaction between hydrogen peroxide and chloride ions.
   c. False Lysozyme is oxygen independent and acts to split peptidoglycan.
   d. True Hydrogen peroxide is formed when superoxide radicals combine with hydrogen ions.
   e. False Cationic proteins are oxygen independent and damage microbial membranes.

7. a. False Natural killer cells do not recognize specific individual antigens, but characteristics of cells such as the level of MHC expression.
   b. True KIRs detect classical MHC class I; CD94:NKG2 detects non-classical MHC class I.
   c. True Natural killer cells can kill antibody-coated cells irrespective of the presence of MHC.
   d. False Natural killer cells are part of the innate immune system and do not exhibit memory.
   e. False Killing is via apoptosis.

8. a. False The classical pathway is activated by antibody bound to antigen.
   b. True The lectin pathway is activated when mannan-binding lectin binds to bacterial carbohydrates.
   c. True The alternative pathway starts with spontaneous activation of C3.
   d. True Complement killing is by formation of the membrane attack complex.
   e. True Complement recruits inflammatory cells and kills or opsonizes pathogens.

9. a. False Factor H prevents assembly of C3 convertase.
   b. False Decay accelerating factor accelerates the decay of C3 convertase.

c. True   Factor I and membrane cofactor protein cleave C3b and C4b.

d. True   CD59 (protectin) prevents formation of the membrane attack complex.

e. True   C1 inhibitor inhibits C1.

10. a. True   The T cell receptor consists of four immunoglobulin domains.

b. False   CD3-ε, γ and δ contain immunoglobulin domains but ζ does not.

c. True   HLA molecules consist of four immunoglobulin domains.

d. True   Certain adhesion molecules, including ICAM-1, are members of the immunoglobulin gene superfamily.

e. True   The polyimmunoglobulin receptor is a member of the immunoglobulin gene superfamily.

11. a. False   T cell maturation occurs in the thymus, therefore it is a primary lymphoid organ.

b. False   Lymph node germinal follicles are primarily composed of B cells.

c. False   Diversity in immunoglobulin molecules is generated in the bone marrow, but somatic hypermutation occurs within germinal centres.

d. False   Lymph nodes sample antigen from lymph (fluid drained from interstitial tissues).

e. True   Peyer's patches are organized mucosal-associated lymphoid organs.

12. a. False   The light chain has only V and J segments.

b. False   Somatic hypermutation of immunoglobulin occurs after encountering antigen.

c. False   T cells do not undergo somatic hypermutation.

d. True   Antibody affinity increases during an immune response because of somatic hypermutation.

e. False   The T cell receptor repertoire depends on HLA molecules, which are polymorphic.

13. a. True   IgA is secreted across mucosal surfaces.
b. True   IgA is also secreted in breast milk.
c. False   IgG is the most abundant immunoglobulin in blood.
d. False   IgG, not IgA, crosses the placenta.
e. True   IgA is usually dimeric.

14. a. True   HLA molecules are human MHC molecules.

b. False   The HLA complex is found on chromosome 6.

c. True   The class III region of HLA encodes C4 and C2.

d. True   The TNF gene is encoded within the MHC.

e. False β_2-microglobulin is not encoded on chromosome 6.

15. a. True   The acute phase plasma proteins increase in concentration.

b. False   Thrombocytosis develops.

c. False   Levels of caeruloplasmin rise to about 150% of normal levels.

d. True   CRP and SAA rise rapidly.

e. False   Plasma viscosity and ESR are raised.

16. a. False   Class I molecules are formed from α-chains and β_2-microglobulin.

b. True $CD8^+$ T cells are class I MHC-restricted, targeting them to endogenous antigen presentation.

c. False   All nucleated cells express class I molecules.

d. True   Class I molecules present endogenous antigen.

e. False   Class I molecules present peptides 9 amino acids long, class II present peptides 12–15 peptides long.

17. a. True   Each immunoglobulin molecule consists of two identical heavy chains and two identical light chains.

b. False   The variable regions of the heavy and light chains are derived from different genetic recombination events.

c. False   The variable regions comprise the antigen-binding site.

d. False   TCR signals through CD3.

e. False   Approximately 5% of T cells express αβ receptors.

18. a. True   Interferons α and β are produced by a wide number of cells to induce an antiviral state (interferon-γ is produced by T cells).

b. False   T cells are part of the adaptive immune response.

c. True   The complement system is a cascade of proteins involved in the innate immune system.

d. False   Antibodies are specific and therefore part of the adaptive response.

e. True   Acute phase proteins are innate molecules.

19. a. True   Malformation of the third and fourth pharyngeal pouches can lead to failure of thymic development.

b. False   In DiGeorge syndrome the thymus is hypoplastic.

c. False The parathyroid glands also fail to develop.

d. True Cardiac defects occur in DiGeorge syndrome.

e. True Recurrent infections occur in DiGeorge syndrome because of the lack of T cells.

20. a. True Complement proteins are proenzymes.

b. False Complement can also be activated by lectins, which bind bacteria.

c. False The alternative pathway is activated spontaneously, particularly on cell surfaces.

d. True The membrane attack complex (MAC) is formed from C5, C6, C7, C8 and C9.

e. True C3 convertase provides a major amplification step.

21. a. False Antigen enters lymph nodes via lymphatics.

b. True Lymph filters from the outside to the inside of the node.

c. True Lymph nodes provide an environment for T and B cell activation.

d. True Lymphocytes leave the blood through high endothelial vessels.

e. False Lymph circulates passively.

22. a. True Pharyngeal tonsils are organized MALT.

b. True The appendix is an organized MALT found in the caecum.

c. False The thymus is a secondary lymphoid organ not associated with the mucosa.

d. True Peyer's patches are organized MALT found throughout the small and large intestine.

e. False Inguinal lymph nodes drain lymph from the lower limbs.

23. a. True The thymus is bilobed.

b. False The thymus is normally found in the mediastinum, but can extend into the neck.

c. True Over 95% of T cell precursors undergo apoptosis in the thymus.

d. False Stromal cells support developing thymocytes.

e. True Thymic epithelial cells produce several hormones that are essential for the differentiation and maturation of thymocytes.

24. a. True T helper cells are usually $CD4^+$.

b. True T cell help is required to produce antibodies against protein antigens.

c. True Cytokines produced by T cells are important in the adaptive and innate immune responses.

d. False T helper cells express TCRs in order to detect MHC class II molecules and antigen on APCs.

e. True Different T helper subsets mediate antibody or cell-mediated responses.

25. a. True Vascular changes and neutrophil infiltration are mediated by several chemical mediators.

b. True TNF-α is one of the important mediators.

c. False Activation of the complement system produces important mediators for acute inflammation.

d. True Coagulation and fibrinolytic systems are also involved in acute inflammation.

e. False ICAM molecules are upregulated on endothelial cells.

26. a. True Adhesion molecules are induced on the endothelium.

b. True Production of platelet-activating factor and prostacyclin is increased.

c. True Neutrophils are attracted by chemotactic cytokines.

d. True Fibroblasts proliferate and increase collagen synthesis.

e. True Cytokines are involved in the development of the acute phase response.

27. a. False PAF is produced from cell membrane phospholipids but not from arachidonic acid.

b. True Leukotriene B_4 is produced from 5-HPETE, a metabolite of arachidonic acid.

c. True Thromboxane A_2 is an endoperoxide produced from the metabolism of arachidonic acid.

d. False Perforin is produced and stored in vesicles in cytotoxic T cells and natural killer cells.

e. True Prostacyclin is an endoperoxide produced from the metabolism of arachidonic acid.

28. a. True Neutrophils are the first cells to sites of inflammation.

b. False L-selectin is constitutively expressed by leucocytes, whereas E- and P-selectin must be induced on endothelial cells.

c. True Integrin molecules are rapidly induced and strengthen binding.

d. True Integrin molecules such as $\alpha_4\beta_7$ are important for leucocyte homing.

e. False Leucocytes change shape to move between endothelial cells.

29. a. False Macrophages and not neutrophils dominate chronic inflammation.

b. True Macrophages are central to chronic inflammation.

c. True Granulomas can result as part of a chronic inflammatory process.

d. True TNF-α is needed for granuloma formation and maintenance.

e. False Lymphocytes are always involved in chronic inflammatory responses.

30. a. True Tissue injury is caused by release of several mediators including toxic oxygen metabolites.

b. False A chronic inflammatory response will persist or result in scar formation.

c. True Systemic features, such as weight loss and persistent fever, are characteristic of chronic inflammation.

d. True Macrophages present antigen to T cells.

e. True Macrophages release fibrogenic cytokines.

31. a. False Lysozyme is an important part of the innate response to bacteria.

b. True Antibodies can bind to free virus, preventing entry to cells and increasing phagocytosis.

c. True Interferons induce antiviral states in uninfected cells and activate macrophages and natural killer cells.

d. False Eosinophils are involved in the response against large extracellular parasites such as helminths.

e. True Cytotoxic T cells recognize virally infected cells and kill them.

32. a. True Some viruses undergo gradual mutation, the new mutant strain causes a fresh epidemic every few years, e.g. influenza.

b. True MHC expression is reduced by several viruses, including CMV, EBV and adenovirus.

c. True Viruses with unstable genomes (e.g. HIV) undergo mutation within the host. The mutated viruses escape the immune system.

d. False Some bacteria release exotoxins. Viral genomes are too small to encode exotoxins.

e. True HSV, EBV and varicella zoster can become latent.

33. a. True Antigenic variation circumvents immunological memory.

b. True Trypanosomes and malaria are immunosuppressive.

c. True Protozoa often have several different stages during infection, thereby presenting several challenges to the immune system.

d. True By infecting intracellularly, humoral immunity is less effective.

e. True Trypanosomes can escape from phagosomes into the cytoplasm.

34. a. False IgE mediates type I reactions.

b. True Complexes composed of antigen and antibody cause type III hypersensitivity.

c. True Mast cell degranulation causes type I hypersensitivity.

d. False Rhesus incompatibility is a type II hypersensitivity reaction.

e. True In the Arthus reaction, immune complexes are deposited in the tissues.

35. a. True The skin-prick test is for type I (allergic) hypersensitivity.

b. True A Mantoux test looks for type IV hypersensitivity against mycobacterium.

c. True Allergic rhinitis is a type I reaction.

d. True Graves' disease is a type II reaction where antibodies stimulate thyroid cell surface TSH receptors.

e. False Rheumatoid arthritis is a hypersensitivity reaction. Osteoarthritis is believed to be a degenerative condition.

36. a. False Paracetamol is not a good anti-inflammatory.

b. False Steroids can be given orally and topically as well as intravenously.

c. False NSAIDs inhibit cyclo-oxygenase.

d. True Anti-TNF-α is a new type of anti-inflammatory drug.

e. True Adverse effects of NSAIDs include nephrotoxicity, bronchospasm and gastrointestinal upset.

37. a. True Allergies are type I immediate reactions. They can become chronic, in which case, IgE is still involved.

b. True In asthma, airway obstruction can be reversed by 15% or more.

c. True Pollen and dust mites are common allergens.

d. True Atopic conditions include hay fever, asthma and atopic eczema.

e. False Anaphylaxis is associated with hypotension and shock.

38. a. True Densensitization consists of controlled exposure to graded doses of allergen.

b. False Antihistamines control the symptoms of allergy but do not cure them.

c. True   Steroids are commonly used in asthma and eczema.

d. True   Intramuscular or intravenous adrenaline is important for the resuscitation of patients with anaphylaxis.

e. True   Many asthmatics can become symptom free by using prophylactic treatment.

39. a. True   Central tolerance in the bone marrow or thymus deletes the most self-reactive lymphocytes.

b. True   Anergic cells do not respond to antigen.

c. False   Molecular mimicry can initiate autoimmunity by breaking self-tolerance.

d. True   Immune privileged sites can express Fas ligand, causing T cells to apoptose and thereby prevent exposure to sequestered antigen.

e. True   Regulatory T cells are important for peripheral tolerance.

40. a. False   SLE is systemic.

b. False   SLE occurs nine times more commonly in women than in men.

c. True   SLE patients produce antibodies which react with anti-double-stranded DNA or ribonucleoproteins.

d. False   SLE is associated with HLA-DR2 or DR3.

e. True   A photosensitive malar 'butterfly' rash is common.

41. a. True   RA is characterized by inflammation of the synovium and destruction of the articular cartilage.

b. False   Inflammation affects many tissues in RA.

c. True   New treatment strategies aim to block the effects of TNF.

d. True   RA occurs three times more commonly in women than in men.

e. False   The precise autoantigen(s) in RA are not defined.

42. a. False   25% of people with RA will not be RF positive.

b. True   Rheumatoid factor is an autoantibody.

c. False   Rheumatoid factor is an IgM antibody directed against IgG.

d. True   Complement activation can occur.

e. True   Rheumatoid factor amplifies the immune response.

43. a. False   Reiter's syndrome is a triad of arthritis, conjunctivitis and urethritis.

b. True   Hashimoto's thyroiditis is a cause of goitrous hypothyroidism.

c. True   Myasthenia gravis results from anti-acetylcholine receptor antibodies.

d. True   Graves' disease results from anti-TSH receptor antibodies.

e. False   Polyarteritis nodosa is an autoimmune disease affecting the vasculature (vasculitis).

44. a. True   It is a primary deficiency in neutrophil killing.

b. True   Transient hypogammaglobulinaemia of infancy occurs if the production of antibody by infants is delayed or if the baby is born prematurely.

c. False   Splenectomy is not a cause of primary immunodeficiency but can result in a predisposition to infection.

d. False   AIDS is a secondary immunodeficiency.

e. True   Wiskott–Aldrich syndrome produces a primary lymphocyte deficiency.

45. a. True   Resulting from chronic bronchial infection.

b. True   Resulting from chronic gastrointestinal tract infection.

c. False   Rheumatoid arthritis is not associated with antibody deficiency.

d. False   Antibody deficiency reduces viscosity.

e. True   Mycoplasma is common in antibody deficiency.

46. a. True   B cells are polyclonally activated in HIV infection.

b. True   T cells become defective.

c. False   Viral replication can be high even during the latent phase of HIV infection.

d. True   Antibodies are generated against gp120 and gp41 but are not effective at clearing infection.

e. True   Lymph nodes become persistently large during HIV infection.

47. a. True   CMV retinitis occurs at CD4 counts below 50.

b. True   *Pneumocystis carinii* pneumonia is common if the CD4 count falls below 200.

c. True   Oesophageal candidiasis is common at CD4 counts below 200.

d. True   *Mycobacterium avium intracellulare* (MAC) is common at CD4 counts below 50.

e. True   Toxoplasmosis is common at CD4 counts below 200.

48. a. False   MMR is given at 12–15 months and again at 4–5 years.

165

b.	True	BCG is given to neonates in at-risk groups or at 10–14 years of age. Some countries do not give BCG routinely, e.g. US.
c.	True	Influenza vaccine is given to at-risk groups, including over-65 year olds.
d.	True	Meningococcal C vaccine is given at 2, 3 and 4 months.
e.	True	Tetanus vaccine requires several boosters.

49.
a.	True	The Sabin vaccine uses live polio; the Salk vaccine is inactivated polio.
b.	False	Tetanus toxoid is used for vaccination.
c.	True	The bacille Calmette–Guérin vaccine is used for tuberculosis.
d.	True	Rubella is a live vaccine.
e.	False	Hepatitis B vaccine uses surface antigen.

50.
a.	False	Hyperacute rejection is rapid because antibodies have been induced prior to transplantation, e.g. by blood transfusion.
b.	False	Acute cellular rejection is mediated by T cells.
c.	False	Preformed antibodies against HLA cause hyperacute rejection.
d.	True	Chronic rejection can be caused by deposition of immune complexes, cell-mediated rejection or viral infection.
e.	True	The complement and clotting cascades are activated in hyperacute rejection.

51.
a.	True	A monozygous twin is genetically identical and should not stimulate the immune system.
b.	True	Steroids are useful anti-inflammatory and immunosuppressive drugs.
c.	True	Antibodies to T cells can reduce the risk of transplant rejection.
d.	True	'Warm ischaemia' is a major risk factor for transplant rejection.
e.	False	Most transplants are more successful if HLA molecules and blood group antigens are matched.

52.
a.	True	Haemopoiesis starts in the bone marrow prior to birth and does not occur elsewhere unless the bone marrow fails to meet the need for new cells.
b.	True	Bone marrow is found throughout the skeleton.
c.	True	Yellow bone marrow is almost entirely fat.
d.	True	Bone marrow macrophages transfer iron to developing red cells, remove debris from haemopoiesis and regulate differentiation and maturation of haemopoietic cells.

e.	True	T lymphocyte precursors are formed in the bone marrow but move to the thymus for maturation.

53.
a.	False	The spleen is posterior to the stomach on the left side of the body.
b.	True	The red pulp removes old or defective erythrocytes and platelets from the circulation.
c.	False	Most of the B cell follicles in the spleen will have been stimulated.
d.	True	The spleen starts developing during the fifth week of fetal life.
e.	True	Primary cancers of the spleen are very rare.

54.
a.	False	Haemopoietic stem cells are found in the liver and spleen, as well as in the bone marrow.
b.	True	They can differentiate into any of the blood cells.
c.	True	Stem cells self-replicate.
d.	True	Stem cells divide to become lineage-committed stem cells.
e.	True	The actions of growth factors allow lineage commitment and differentiation.

55.
a.	True	Congestive splenomegaly is due to venous congestion.
b.	False	In the UK, splenomegaly is most commonly due to haematological disorders.
c.	True	Splenic infarction occurs in myeloproliferative disorders and sickle-cell disease.
d.	True	EBV infection, trauma and haemopoietic disorders can cause splenic rupture.
e.	True	The spleen can become enlarged due to lymphomas and leukaemias.

56.
a.	True	The spleen is removed to stop blood loss.
b.	True	Splenic tumours are an indication for splenectomy.
c.	True	Idiopathic thrombocytopenic purpura can be treated by splenectomy.
d.	True	Haemolytic anaemias can be improved by splenectomy.
e.	True	Splenic cysts are an indication for splenectomy.

57.
a.	True	Hereditary spherocytosis is an autosomal dominant condition due to inheritance of a defective spectrin gene.
b.	False	Leads to extravascular haemolysis.
c.	True	Spherocytes are seen in the peripheral blood.
d.	True	Spherocytes lyse in less hypotonic solutions than normal red cells.

e. False   Spherocytes lyse readily on incubation at 37°C (autohaemolysis).

58. a. True   In β-thalassaemia major a severe microcytic, hypochromic anaemia is seen.

b. True   Iron overload is caused by increased enteric absorption and regular blood transfusions.

c. False   Most red blood cells are destroyed in the marrow; those that reach the circulation have a shortened lifespan.

d. True   β-thalassaemia major is due to two defective copies of the β-chain gene.

e. False   HbA is not present on electrophoresis.

59. a. False   Erythrocytes are not nucleated.

b. True   They are derived from the CFU-GEMM along with granulocytes, macrophages and megakaryocytes.

c. True   Their primary function is the transport of O_2 and CO_2.

d. False   The normal lifespan is 120 days.

e. False   They have a biconcave discoid shape.

60. a. False   Iron is actively absorbed in the duodenum and jejunum.

b. False   There is no mechanism to excrete excess iron.

c. False   Iron is transported in the blood bound to transferrin (it is stored with apoferritin).

d. True   Primary haemochromatosis is an autosomal recessive disorder characterized by excessive intestinal absorption of iron.

e. False   Total body stores of iron are ~4 g.

61. a. False   Adult haemoglobin is composed of two α-chains with either two β- or two δ-chains.

b. True   Oxygen is transported by haemoglobin bound to haem.

c. True   Increased H^+ concentration causes the oxygen dissociation curve to shift to the right—the Bohr effect.

d. True   Oxygen binding follows a sigmoidal curve due to allosteric interactions between the subunits.

e. False   2,3-Diphosphoglycerate levels rise during hypoxia to increase the release of oxygen at the tissues.

62. a. False   Vitamin B_{12} is absorbed in the terminal ileum after combining with intrinsic factor produced in the stomach.

b. True   It is composed of cobalamin (cobalt containing) bound to a methyl or adenosyl group.

c. True   Absorption is reduced after total gastrectomy due to a lack of intrinsic factor.

d. False   Requires intrinsic factor for absorption.

e. False   It cannot be synthesized by the body.

63. a. True   Folic acid is found primarily in green vegetables.

b. False   Folic acid is absorbed in the duodenum and jejunum.

c. False   The daily requirement is 100–200 µg.

d. True   Deficiency can be caused by malabsorption in coeliac disease.

e. False   During pregnancy, folic acid requirement is increased, and supplements are often given to prevent neural tube defects in the fetus.

64. a. False   Iron deficiency causes a microcytic anaemia.

b. True   Tuberculosis causes a normochromic, normocytic anaemia of chronic disease.

c. True   Rheumatoid arthritis causes a normochromic, normocytic anaemia of chronic disease.

d. False   Vitamin B_{12} causes a macrocytic anaemia.

e. False   Thalassaemia causes a microcytic anaemia.

65. a. True   Glossitis is a feature of iron-deficiency anaemia.

b. True   Koilonychia is a feature specific to iron-deficiency anaemia.

c. False   The anaemia produced is microcytic.

d. True   It is distinguished from thalassaemia and anaemia of chronic disease by a low serum iron and ferritin.

e. False   Serum transferrin is increased in iron deficiency.

66. a. True   Polycythaemia rubra vera is a primary cause of polycythaemia.

b. False   Dehydration causes a relative polycythaemia.

c. True   Renal carcinoma causes an absolute polycythaemia due to increased erythropoietin.

d. True   Cyanotic heart disease causes an absolute polycythaemia due to increased erythropoietin.

e. False   Diuretic therapy causes a relative polycythaemia.

67. a. True   Pronormoblasts are erythrocyte precursors.

b. True   Normoblasts are erythrocyte precursors.

c. False   Stomatocytes are seen in liver disease and in alcoholism.

d. True   Reticulocytes are erythrocyte precursors.

e. False   Echinocytes are seen in renal disease.

68. a. True   Pigment gallstones are due to excess bilirubin from the breakdown of protoporphyrin.

b. False   Plasma haptoglobin falls because it binds to the free haemoglobin in the blood.

c. True   Haemosiderin is excreted in the urine.

d. True   Release of haemoglobin from lysed erythrocytes.

e. True   Excess reticulocytes enter the blood in an effort to increase red cell mass.

69. a. True   Infection is an oxidizing factor associated with haemolysis when there is a lack of reduced glutathione.

b. False   Acidosis, e.g. diabetic ketoacidosis, precipitates haemolysis.

c. True   Primaquine is an oxidizing factor associated with haemolysis when there is a lack of reduced glutathione.

d. True   Fava beans are oxidizing factors associated with haemolysis when there is a lack of reduced glutathione.

e. False   The circulation should be supported during an acute crisis.

70. a. True   Pneumococcal, meningococcal and Hib vaccine are routinely given to patients with sickle-cell anaemia.

b. True   Folic acid is given due to an increased rate of erythropoiesis.

c. True   Penicillin prophylaxis and antibiotics for prompt treatment of infections are commonly used.

d. True   Blood or exchange transfusions can be given to maintain an adequate haemoglobin level.

e. True   Fluids are often needed in the management of acute crises.

71. a. True   It has a sigmoidal oxygen dissociation curve.

b. False   Has a higher affinity for oxygen than adult haemoglobin.

c. True   It may persist in β-thalassaemia in order to increase the oxygen carrying capacity of blood.

d. True   It is produced in the fetal liver and spleen.

e. False   Fetal haemoglobin is composed of two α- and two γ-chains.

72. a. True   Erythropoietin is required for red-cell maturation, where it prevents red-cell precursors from undergoing apoptosis.

b. False   The kidneys are the principal source of erythropoietin.

c. True   The major stimulus for release is hypoxia.

d. True   Recombinant erythropoietin is indicated for use in a number of clinical diseases.

e. False   Required for red-cell maturation.

73. a. True   It can be caused by drugs, irradiation and chemicals; 50% are idiopathic.

b. True   It may be part of a congenital syndrome.

c. True   It may be associated with acute viral infection.

d. False   Aplastic anaemia is a pancytopenia resulting from aplastic bone marrow.

e. True   Androgens are used to treat aplastic anaemia.

74. a. True   Prosthetic heart valves can cause fragmentation of red cells.

b. True   Acute renal failure is a feature of intravascular haemolysis.

c. False   Bilirubin is not found in urine because it is bound to albumin.

d. True   Increased urobilinogen is common.

e. False   The anaemia is normo- or macrocytic.

75. a. False   Polymorphonuclear leucocytes (neutrophils) have a multilobed nucleus.

b. False   They respond primarily to bacterial infection.

c. True   They have a granular cytoplasm.

d. True   They are phagocytic.

e. True   They are a major constituent of pus.

76. a. True   Myelodysplastic syndromes are acquired bone marrow neoplasias.

b. False   Are due to defects in myeloid precursors.

c. True   They slowly progress to acute myeloid leukaemia.

d. False   Most commonly occur in elderly men.

e. True   Prognosis is worst in those with high levels of marrow blasts (>5%).

77. a. True   Leucostatic symptoms occur in leukaemias.

b. False   They are caused by white-cell thrombi.

c. True   They do include retinal haemorrhage.

d. True   They do include a reduced level of consciousness.

e. False   They resolve if the white-cell count decreases.

78. a. True   Superficial, asymmetric, painless lymphadenopathy is consistent with a diagnosis of non-Hodgkin's lymphoma.

b. False — Reed–Sternberg cells are pathognomonic of Hodgkin's disease.

c. True — Fever, night sweats and weight loss are all features of non-Hodgkin's lymphoma.

d. True — Non-Hodgkin's lymphoma is associated with inherited disorders such as Fanconi's syndrome.

e. True — Non-Hodgkin's lymphoma is associated with immunodeficiency, e.g. HIV or immunosuppressive therapy.

79. a. True — Polycythaemia rubra vera is a myeloproliferative disorder.

b. False — Sideroblastic anaemia is a myelodysplastic syndrome.

c. True — Myelofibrosis is a myeloproliferative disorder.

d. True — Primary thrombocythaemia is a myeloproliferative disorder.

e. False — Acute lymphoblastic leukaemia is a disease of lymphoid not myeloid lineage.

80. a. True — Macrophages are differentiated monocytes found in the tissues.

b. True — Their primary roles include phagocytosis.

c. True — They play an important role in the adaptive immune response.

d. True — They may be infected by HIV.

e. False — Macrophages are not important in allergic responses (mast cells).

81. a. True — Chronic lymphocytic leukaemia accounts for 20–50% of leukaemias.

b. False — It is a slowly progressive condition.

c. True — 95% are B cell in origin.

d. True — Autoimmune haemolytic anaemias are common.

e. False — It never converts to an acute leukaemia.

82. a. True — Acute lymphoblastic leukaemia is the most common leukaemia in childhood and is rare in adults.

b. True — The best prognosis is between the ages of 2 and 10.

c. False — Remission rates of over 70% are seen.

d. False — 80% of cases are B cell in origin.

e. True — Aetiological factors include radiation, chemicals, Down syndrome and Fanconi's syndrome.

83. a. False — Acute myeloblastic leukaemia is an accumulation of primitive myeloblasts in the bone marrow and peripheral blood.

b. True — It is associated with hereditary abnormalities such as Down syndrome.

c. False — It can be due to a variety of chromosomal rearrangements (isochromosome 12p is associated with testicular tumours).

d. False — Only 15% of over-60 year olds are cured.

e. True — Patients are often unwell at presentation and can have a bleeding disorder.

84. a. True — Chronic myeloid leukaemia is usually identified in the chronic phase, either incidentally or due to constitutional or leucostatic symptoms.

b. False — >90% of patients progress to an accelerated phase or blast crisis within 10 years.

c. True — The Philadelphia chromosome—t(9;22)—is identified in more than 90% of cases.

d. True — The Philadelphia chromosome is the target for the tyrosine kinase inhibitor Glivec.

e. True — Bone marrow transplantation is potentially curative but is not commonly used.

85. a. False — Monoclonal light chains are produced in large quantity and are excreted in urine, where they are known as Bence Jones protein.

b. True — Neurological lesions occur due to vertebral collapse.

c. True — An acquired hypogammaglobulinaemia and neutropenia leads to repeated infection.

d. True — It causes multiple osteolytic bone lesions.

e. True — Multiple myeloma is a malignant proliferation of plasma cells, which make up more than 10% of bone marrow cells.

86. a. True — Aplastic anaemia is a cause of generalized marrow failure.

b. True — Leukaemia is also a cause of generalized marrow failure.

c. True — Kostmann's syndrome is a congenital defect resulting in neutropenia.

d. True — Causes generalized marrow suppression.

e. True — Several different drugs, including chloroquine, can lead to a neutropenia.

87. a. False — Platelets are derived from megakaryocyte cytoplasm.

b. False — Platelet adhesion or aggregation requires von Willebrand's factor.

c. True — They form a primary platelet plug to slow bleeding.

169

d. True   Platelets interact with type I, II and III collagen via GPIa.

e. False Aggregation is enhanced by thromboxane A_2 and inhibited by prostacyclin.

88. a. True   Many drugs can cause increased bleeding, including marrow suppressants and anticoagulants.

b. True   Chemo- and radiotherapy cause bleeding by damage to tissues and reduction in platelets due to marrow suppression.

c. True   Haemophila A and B are X-linked.

d. True   Splenomegaly leads to increased sequestration and destruction of platelets.

e. True   Defective platelets cannot form the primary haemostatic plug.

89. a. True   Factor II (prothrombin) is a vitamin-K-dependent clotting factor.

b. True   Factor IX is a vitamin-K-dependent clotting factor.

c. False Vitamin K acts by allowing post-translational γ-carboxylation of glutamic acid residues.

d. True   It is a fat-soluble vitamin and deficiency can result from fat malabsorption.

e. False Haemophilia A is caused by a factor VIII deficiency.

90. a. True   The prothrombin time is increased in disseminated intravascular coagulation.

b. False In von Willebrand's disease bleeding time is extended and activated partial thromboplastin time may be prolonged.

c. True   The prothrombin time is increased in vitamin K deficiency.

d. False Activated partial thromboplastin time is increased in haemophilia A but the prothrombin time is normal.

e. False Activated partial thromboplastin time is increased in haemophilia B but the prothrombin time is normal.

91. a. True   Factor V Leiden is less sensitive to inactivation by protein C and therefore confers an increased risk of clotting.

b. True   Disseminated cancers secrete substances that activate factor X.

c. True   Oestrogen therapy increases levels of the vitamin-K-dependent factors and lowers antithrombin III and tissue plasminogen activator levels.

d. True   Protein C inhibits factors V and VIII and enhances fibrinolysis, therefore a deficiency increases the risk of clotting.

e. True   Prolonged immobilization causes venous stasis and clotting.

92. a. False Idiopathic thrombocytopenic purpura (ITP) is caused by either antibody–viral-antigen complexes or anti-platelet IgG autoantibodies.

b. True   IgG anti-platelet antibodies are found in the plasma.

c. True   It occurs in disorders causing an aberrant immune response such as HIV disease.

d. True   High-dose glucocorticoids are used in ITP to suppress the abnormal immune response.

e. False Fresh-frozen plasma will not raise the platelet count.

93. a. False Heparin is given intravenously or subcutaneously.

b. False Standard heparin is monitored by activated partial thromboplastin time (APTT); low-molecular-weight heparin does not need APTT monitoring.

c. True   Heparin is a glycosaminoglycan.

d. True   At different molecular weights the activity of heparin is different, with lower-molecular-weight heparins having greater activity against factor Xa than standard heparin.

e. False Heparin (mucopolysaccharide) and warfarin (coumarin or indandione derivatives) are not structurally related.

94. a. True   Proteins C and S inhibit clotting factors V and VIII and enhance fibrinolysis.

b. False Plasminogen activator inhibitors prevent fibrinolysis by plasmin.

c. True   Reduced levels of platelets diminish clotting.

d. True   Streptokinase is a fibrinolytic agent.

e. False Christmas factor (factor IX) is part of the coagulation cascade.

95. a. False Haemophilia A is X-linked.

b. False Haemophilia A is not associated with social class.

c. False Treated prophylactically with factor VIII.

d. True   Repeated bleeds into joints result in deformity.

e. True   It is caused by factor VIII deficiency and so may be mimicked by von Willebrand's disease (pseudohaemophilia).

96. a. True   The normal haemoglobin for a male is 13–17 g/dL.

b. True   Normal white cell count is $4–10 \times 10^9$/L.

c. True pO_2 is normally 100 mmHg in arterial blood, although 40 mmHg is the normal level in mixed venous blood.

d. False   Reticulocytes should account for only 1–2% of peripheral red blood cells.

e. False   Normal platelet levels are 150–400 × 10^9/L.

97. a. True   Howell–Jolly bodies are inclusions in red cells seen on a peripheral blood smear after splenectomy.

b. True   Auer rods are inclusions in white cells seen on a peripheral blood smear of a patient with AML.

c. False   Philadelphia chromosome is detected by cytogenetic techniques.

d. True   Reticulocytosis may be detected.

e. False   Bence Jones protein is found only in urine.

98. a. False   People who are blood group O can have parents who are both group O, although parents who are heterozygous for group A or B can pass on an O allele.

b. True   Group A people will produce anti-B antibodies.

c. False   In blood group O it is the H antigen that is left unchanged.

d. False   Group AB is the universal recipient and group O the universal donor.

e. False   Anti-ABO antibodies are IgM leading to intravascular haemolysis.

99. a. True   Rhesus D incompatibility is a common cause of haemolytic disease of the newborn.

b. False   It does not usually occur in the first child because the mother has not previously been sensitized to the rhesus D antigen.

c. False   Rhesus D is not the only cause of haemolytic disease of the newborn.

d. True   Passive immunization can prevent the mother producing antibodies.

e. False   The antibodies are IgG.

100. a. True   Donor red cells are destroyed by IgM antibodies in the recipient's serum.

b. True   IgM antibodies can fix complement.

c. False   Symptoms occur within minutes to hours.

d. False   Hypo- not hypertension occurs, but the other symptoms are present.

e. True   Release of tissue thromboplastin from lysed red cells can lead to disseminated intravascular coagulation.

1. Refer to Fig. 1.30, p. 28.

2. Positive and negative selection of T cells occurs during T cell maturation in the thymus. Positive selection of T cells refers to the process whereby T cells that are capable of binding self-major histocompatibility complex (MHC) molecules are selected for. It involves the interaction of developing $CD4^+ CD8^+$ T cells with thymic epithelial cells that express high levels of class I and class II molecules. T cells that do not interact with MHC undergo apoptosis. This is because they do not receive a protective signal as a result of the interaction between the T cell receptor (TCR) and MHC.

   Some of the T cells that survive positive selection have receptors with high affinity for self-MHC and self-antigen. These $CD4^+ CD8^+$ T cells undergo negative selection. Negative selection is thought to be mediated by dendritic cells (which are derived from the bone marrow). These cells express high levels of class I and class II MHC molecules, which interact with T cells expressing high-affinity receptors for self-MHC alone or self-MHC and antigen. These 'self-reactive' T cells are, therefore, removed via apoptosis.

   The positive and negative selection processes result in a population of thymocytes that can bind self-MHC at low affinity but are not stimulated by self-MHC plus self-antigen. Positive selection occurs in the cortex of the thymus. Negative selection occurs in the corticomedullary junction and medulla of the thymus.

3. Refer to Fig. 4.9, p. 80.

4. The structure of an Ig molecule is shown in Fig. 1.22. The functions are:
   - Complement fixation
   - Opsonization
   - Neutralization of toxins
   - Participation in antibody-dependent cell-mediated cytotoxicity
   - Protection of the neonate (IgG crossing the placenta and IgA in breast milk)
   - Mast cell activation in parasitic infestations (IgE).

5. Pernicious anaemia is a chronic atrophic gastritis with a probable autoimmune aetiology. It is the most common cause of vitamin B_{12} deficiency in adults. Autoantibodies directed against both the gastric parietal cells and intrinsic factor (IF) are detectable in the serum and gastric juice of most patients. Damage to the parietal cells and failure of formation and absorption of the B_{12}–IF complex result.

   Achlorhydria is an accompanying feature (parietal cells are also responsible for secreting H^+). Pernicious anaemia is associated with autoimmune thyroid disease and patients are at an increased risk of gastric carcinoma. Clinical features include:
   - A lemon-yellow colour to the skin, caused by a combination of pallor and jaundice resulting from ineffective erythropoiesis
   - Glossitis
   - Gastrointestinal disturbances
   - Weight loss
   - Neurological abnormalities (peripheral neuropathy, subacute degeneration of the spinal cord involving the posterior and lateral columns, and psychiatric disturbances).

   The diagnosis is made by either demonstrating the presence of antibodies to intrinsic factor in the patient's serum or by using the Schilling test.

6. Haemolytic disease of the newborn is the result of the passage of IgG antibodies from the maternal circulation across the placenta into the fetal circulation, where they react with fetal red cells and lead to their destruction by the fetal reticuloendothelial system (RES). Haemolytic disease of the newborn can result when a rhesus-negative woman becomes pregnant with a rhesus-positive fetus. During the first pregnancy, the mother is usually sensitized during childbirth, when small amounts of fetal blood leak into the maternal circulation. The mother mounts an antibody response directed against the rhesus antigens. During subsequent pregnancies with a rhesus-positive fetus, IgG antibodies cross the placenta and bind to fetal red cells, resulting in haemolysis. Most cases are due to anti-D antibodies. The most severe consequence is hydrops fetalis.

   Prevention is by intramuscular administration of anti-D IgG to the rhesus-negative mother at 28 weeks and within 72 hours of birth. The D surface antigen on fetal red blood cells in the maternal circulation is coated, thereby preventing a maternal immune response. The rhesus-positive red-blood-cell–anti-D-antibody complex is then removed in the maternal RES.

   Haemolytic disease of the newborn can also be caused by other red blood cell incompatibilities, e.g. Kell or Duffy antigens.

7. Innate immunity comprises the non-specific mechanisms that exist prior to exposure to antigen

and are not altered on repeated exposure to a particular antigen. The immune system provides a rapid, non-specific response.

Adaptive immunity is characterized by specificity and memory. Specificity refers to the ability of the adaptive immune response to distinguish minor differences between antigens. Memory refers to the fact that, once the adaptive immune system has responded to an antigen, it responds more rapidly and to a greater degree upon subsequent exposures, but is still slower than the innate system.

An antigen is any molecule that can be recognized by the adaptive immune system.

An immunogen is a molecule that evokes an immune response. All immunogens are antigenic, but not all antigens are immunogenic.

A hapten is a small antigen that is not immunogenic unless coupled to a larger (usually protein) carrier molecule.

An epitope antigenic determinant (or immunologically active portion of antigen) is the discrete area of the antigen that is recognized by the adaptive immune system.

8. Refer to Fig. 2.29, p. 58.

9. Factors II, VII, IX and X, and proteins C and S are dependent on vitamin K for post-translational modification (see Fig. 6.11, p. 118).

Vitamin K acts as a cofactor for the carboxylase enzyme, resulting in γ-carboxylation of glutamic acid residues, enabling them to bind calcium and, therefore, form complexes with the platelet phospholipid membrane.

In the absence of vitamin K, factors II, VII, IX and X do not undergo γ-carboxylation, cannot bind calcium and are unable to attach onto platelet phospholipid membranes. Consequently, they are activated much more slowly and negligible levels of prothrombin are converted to thrombin.

10. Refer to Fig. 6.1 (p. 112) to answer this question.

11. a. Tuberculosis complicating HIV infection.
b. The finding may have been incidental, e.g. when donating blood, or a person who is at risk, e.g. intravenous drug abuser or sex worker, may have sought an HIV test. In both cases the person may be asymptomatic or have had a mild flu-like illness. Other presenting features may include: skin—molluscum contagiosum; mouth—oral hairy leucoplakia, oral candidiasis, Kaposi's sarcoma; haematological—immune-mediated thrombocytopenic purpura; infections—meningitis (cryptococcal), pneumonia, sinusitis, recurrent gastrointestinal infections (Salmonella, Cryptosporidium, Isospora belli).
c. The underlying condition can be treated with antiretrovirals. They can act at different points within the viral lifecycle.

12. a. Chronic lymphocytic leukaemia.
b. Demonstrate the classical immunophenotypic features of the blood lymphocytes.
c. Because the disease is slowly progressive and of a low grade, chemotherapy or stem cell therapy is used to limit rather than cure the disease. The median survival is 5–8 years.

13. a. Multiple myeloma.
b. • Normochromic normocytic anaemia, resulting from marrow infiltration.
   • Repeated infections. These can occur due to hypogammaglobulinaemia and neutropenia.
   • Hypercalcaemia, which occurs in 10% of cases. This is due to increased reabsorption of bone and is indicative of advanced disease.
   • Chronic renal failure, which occurs in 20–30% of patients. Factors that can contribute to renal failure in multiple myeloma are:
     – increased blood viscosity
     – hypercalcaemia
     – renal tubular obstruction by proteinaceous casts
     – toxic effect of Bence Jones protein on proximal renal tubules
     – infection
     – dehydration
     – non-steroidal anti-inflammatory drugs
     – light-chain deposition in glomeruli.
   • Amyloidosis. This can lead to nephrotic syndrome. An abnormal bleeding tendency occurs owing to the adverse effect of paraprotein on platelets and to coagulation factors.

14. a. Antibody deficiency.
b. Replacement immunoglobulin in the form of pooled human immunoglobulin.

15. Following splenectomy, the patient should be encouraged to mobilize as soon as possible because he is at high risk of thrombosis. He should be made aware that he will have a lifelong increased risk of infection, particularly from encapsulated organisms, e.g. Neisseria meningitides, Streptococcus pneumoniae, Haemophilus influenzae. The following steps should be taken:
• Pneumococcal vaccine should be given, with boosters every 5–10 years.
• Hib and meningococcal vaccine should also be given.
• Prophylactic antibiotics (penicillin) should be given for life.
• He should be given antibiotics that he must take immediately if any symptoms of infection develop.
• He should be warned that tropical infections, e.g. malaria, are more likely to be severe.
• Urgent hospital admission if infection develops.

16. a. Open lung biopsy. This diagnostic test aims to make a histological diagnosis.

    b. Lymphoma, diffuse carcinoma. This patient had a B cell lymphoma.

---

17. a. Concentrated factor VIII or IX (depending on the type of haemophilia), fresh-frozen plasma or blood (if severe blood loss).

    b. Acute HIV seroconversion.

    In the UK, blood products are now routinely tested for HIV antibodies but this might not be the case in developing countries.

---

18. a. Favism.

    b. Negative bilirubin, high urobilinogen and positive haemoglobin (strongly positive for blood with no red cells seen on microscopy).

    c. Reduced haemoglobin (which might be very low, e.g. 4 g/dL) and increased unconjugated bilirubin. Characteristic blood film changes.

---

19. a. A full blood count to ascertain the haemoglobin level in view of the ruddy complexion. In addition, you wish to know the white-cell count and platelet count.

    b. Exclude secondary reasons for a raised haemoglobin, e.g. hypoxia. Confirm an increase in red-cell mass and demonstrate the characteristic bone marrow and clinical features of PRV.

    c. Venesection to reduce blood viscosity. May need the use of cytotoxic therapy, e.g. hydroxyurea.

---

20. a. Anaphylactic response to the bee sting.

    b. The initial management of anaphylaxis is that of resuscitation (airway, breathing, circulation). Adrenaline (epinephrine) should be given intramuscularly and repeated after 5 minutes if there is no improvement. Adrenaline can be given intravenously in life-threatening profound shock or airway obstruction. Fluids might be needed if she is in shock and a β_2-adrenoreceptor agonist can be used to reverse bronchospasm. She should be given adrenaline (EpiPen) to carry with her, so that it can be administered rapidly in an emergency. She should also have a Medic Alert bracelet. She may undergo venom desensitization.

1. Concerning complement:

1. G The membrane attack complex is a set of complement proteins which, on stimulation of the complement cascade, form a polymer that destroys pathogens by punching holes in the cell membrane.

2. I The classical pathway is a rapid complement activation pathway, initiated by the presence of antibody.

3. F C1 esterase inhibitor is deficient in patients with hereditary angioedema.

4. E Anaphylotoxin stimulates the release of histamine, which causes increased vascular permeability and attracts white blood cells to the site of infection.

5. J The processes involved in the complement cascade are regulated by complement inhibitors.

2. Concerning immunization:

1. H An adjuvant is a substance added to vaccines which provides a danger signal to the innate immune system through the stimulation of low grade inflammation.

2. F Active immunity is an immune response produced by the presence of antigen in vaccines.

3. G Clonal expansion of B and T lymphocytes in vaccination produces memory cells, which are activated in a secondary immune response. As a result, the secondary immune response is stronger, occurs faster and lasts longer than the primary.

4. A The transfer of immunoglobulin from one individual to another is termed passive immunity.

5. D A subunit vaccine requires an adjuvant to improve the immune response.

3. Concerning cell surface molecules:

1. G Antigens are substances specifically recognized by receptors of the adaptive immune system.

2. J Collectins are a family of pattern recognition molecules that recognize and opsonize pathogens in solution.

3. C MHC class I recognizes antigen from intracellular pathogens.

4. E Intracellular or phagocytosed antigens expressed simultaneously with MHC are recognized by the T cell receptor on the surface of T lymphocytes.

5. B Toll-like receptors are a family of related molecules found on mammalian cell surfaces; they activate the innate immune system after exposure to a pathogen.

4. Concerning immunoglobins:

1. G Class switch allows different types of immunoglobulin to be produced by individual B cells. During class switch, the heavy chains are switched while retaining the same variable chain.

2. A IgA is an immunoglobulin which is adapted to be secreted across mucosal surfaces.

3. E Type I hypersensitivity is the immune response stimulated by the presence of allergens, a process mediated by IgE.

4. D During class switch, all immunoglobins are derived from molecules of IgM produced by B lymphocytes.

5. C The reaction of ABO antigens and antibodies in the bloodstream is type II hypersensitivity.

5. Concerning B and T lymphocytes:

1. F   In order to become fully active and begin releasing antibody, B cells must be stimulated by T helper cells.

2. J   B and T cells originate from lymphoid stem cells in the bone marrow.

3. C   Plasma cells are a mature type of B lymphocyte. They contain vast amounts of endoplasmic reticulum in order to produce a large quantity of immunoglobulin.

4. A   CD8 is a cell surface marker expressed on cytotoxic T cells.

5. G   Cytotoxic T cells recognize antigen in conjunction with molecules of MHC class I.

6. Concerning anaemia:

1. F   Aplastic anaemia arises from a reduction in the number and function of bone marrow stem cells.

2. J   Iron-deficiency anaemia occurs frequently in women of reproductive age as iron is lost during menstruation as a component of haemoglobin, the red pigment found in red blood cells.

3. G   The cause of vitamin B_{12} deficiency can be diagnosed using the Schilling test.

4. E   Pernicious anaemia can present as chronic atrophic gastritis; it has a probable autoimmune aetiology.

5. H   Sickle cell anaemia is an inherited condition in which red blood cells become elongated into a rigid shape.

7. Concerning haematological investigations:

1. H   The different stages of haemopoiesis can be seen by analysis of a bone marrow smear.

2. D   A differential white count identifies specific levels of neutrophils, lymphocytes, monocytes, eosinophils and basophils in the blood.

3. E   Erythrocyte sedimentation rate (ESR) measures the rate of fall of a column of red blood cells in plasma over 1 hour.

4. B   The function of the coagulation cascade can be assessed by measuring the prothrombin time (PT), a measure of the time it takes for blood to clot.

5. A   Cytogenetic analysis involves the study of the structure and function of chromosomes. This allows any abnormalities to be highlighted and hence can lead to the diagnosis of certain conditions.

8. Concerning red blood cells:

1. E   Erythropoietin is a highly glycosylated polypeptide hormone. Its stimulation causes the differentiation and maturation of erythrocytes.

2. A   Red blood cells contain a red pigment, haemoglobin, which binds and transports oxygen and carbon dioxide. It is composed of two α-chains, with either two β- or two δ-chains.

3. C   The breakdown of red blood cells by macrophages produces bilirubin, which is conjugated in the liver and then excreted in bile.

4. I   Immature red blood cells present in the bone marrow and bloodstream are termed reticulocytes.

5. B   Erythropoiesis is the process by which red blood cells are produced in the bone marrow.

9. Concerning white blood cells:

1. C   Monocytes are precursors of macrophages; they are large, circulating white blood cells, with distinctive, kidney-shaped nuclei.

2. A   Chronic myeloid leukaemia is a myeloproliferative disorder resulting from the proliferation of multipotent myeloid stem cells.

3. D   The first cells recruited to a site of acute inflammation are neutrophils, which are drawn to the area by chemotaxis.

4. G   The delayed stage of type I hypersensitivity is mediated by eosinophils.

5. H   Hodgkin's disease is a condition characterized by the presence of pathognomonic Reed–Sternberg cells or derivatives, typically mixed with a variable inflammatory infiltrate.

10. Concerning haemostasis:

1. G   Thrombin is an enzyme present during the final stages of the coagulation cascade; it converts fibrinogen to fibrin.

2. H   Warfarin is a vitamin K antagonist and therefore inhibits blood clotting.

3. A   The intrinsic clotting pathway takes place entirely within the bloodstream.

4. E   Thrombocytopenia is a decrease in the number of platelets in the blood, resulting in a decreased ability to clot and the potential for increased bleeding.

5. F   The extrinsic clotting pathway is stimulated by tissue factor (TF), a glycoprotein present on fibroblasts.

A

abetalipoproteinaemia, 135
ABO antigens, 127–8, 154
acanthocyte, 135
acetylsalicylic acid, 43–4, 116
achlorhydria, 86
acid hydrolases, 10
acquired immunodeficiency syndrome (AIDS), 55–7
acrocyanosis, 93
actin, 83
activated partial thromboplastin time (APTT), 120,
    122, 142, 143
activation, platelet, 112
active immunization, 58–60
acute cellular graft rejection, 60, 61
acute lymphoblastic leukaemia (ALL), 101, 105, 135,
    153
acute myeloblastic leukaemia (AML), 101, 104, 135,
    153
acute phase proteins (APPs), 9–11, 142–3, 148
ADAMTS-13, 115
adaptive immune system, 3, 4, 20–30
    cell-mediated immunity see cell-mediated immunity
    components of, 5
    humoral immunity see humoral immunity
adenoids, 25
adenosine deaminase (ADA), 54
adenosine diphosphate (ADP), 112
adenovirus, 36
adhesion, platelet, 111, 112, 113
adrenaline, 47, 55–7
adult haemoglobin, 140
adventitial reticular cells, 67
affinity maturation, 19–20
afibrinogenaemia, 142
agammaglobulinaemia, 53
agglutination, 24, 44, 128
aggregation, platelet, 111, 112–13
agranulocytosis, 109–10
AIDS (Acquired immunodeficiency syndrome), 55–7
alcohol, folate deficiency, 87
alleles, 15
allergens, 45, 46, 47
allergic responses, 9
allergies, 39–40, 45–7, 150
allogeneic grafts, 60, 93
alloimmune haemolytic anaemias, 93
alternative pathway, complement, 12, 24
    extracellular bacteria, 37

Alzheimer's disease, 109
amyloid, 109
amyloidosis, 109
anaemia, 85–6, 158
    aplastic, 95, 109, 113, 141, 152
    blood loss, 92–5
    of chronic disease, 94
    Cooley's, 91
    erythrocyte sedimentation rate (ESR), 141
    haemolytic see haemolytic anaemia
    impaired red-cell production, 86–8
    iron-deficiency see iron-deficiency anaemia
    megaloblastic, 86–7, 109, 135, 141
    pernicious, 52, 86–7
    sideroblastic, 88
anaphylatoxins, 37
anaphylaxis, 47
    systemic, 40, 46
angioedema, hereditary, 13
anisocytosis, 135
ankyrin, 83
Ann Arbor staging, 107, 108
antibodies
    diversity, 19
    extracellular bacteria, 37
    primary deficiencies, 53
    production of, 20
    structure and function of, 21–2
    viral infection, 35
antibody-dependent cell-mediated cytotoxicity
        (ADCC), 8, 20, 24, 66
    antibody-mediated (type II) hypersensitivity, 40
    viral infection, 35
antibody-mediated red-cell destruction, 93
antibody-mediated (type II) hypersensitivity, 40–1, 49
anticoagulation, 119–20
antigen-binding region, 22
antigenic drift, 36
antigenic shift, 36
antigenic variation, 36
antigen-presenting cells (APCs), 28, 29
antigens
    processing and presentation of, 17
    receptor diversity, generation, 17–20, 148
    recognition of, 14–15
    red-cell, 93, 127–9
    superantigens, 30
    T-cell-dependent, 20, 21
    T-cell-independent, 20, 21